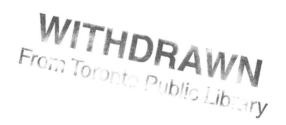
Project Care

Health Care Case Studies, Multimedia, and Projects for Practicing English

Steve Quann
Diana Satin

Ann Arbor
University of Michigan Press

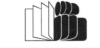

WORLD EDUCATION

Copublished with World Education, Inc.

Acknowledgments

This project grew out of our desire to support our ESOL students who might have family or friends going through the health issues contained in this book. We thank all those who have helped teach us how to better care for others: our parents, our teachers, and our students.

Special thanks to Simone Charpentier, Keiko Mizuguchi, Leonid Newhouse, and David Satin for offering their professional opinions, and for sharing their expertise and insight.

We are fortunate to have as friends two fine writers, P. Carey Reid and Linda Werbner. We want to thank them for sharing their tips of the trade and giving guidance on writing the case studies. Thanks go to Silja Kallenbach, Sabrina Kurtz-Rossi, Julie McKinney, John Strucker and Cynthia Zafft for giving feedback, ideas, and encouragement.

We are deeply grateful for the opportunity to work on this exciting new approach. We have been thinking about linking a book with multimedia and the Internet for a long time. Thanks to Lenore Balliro and Carey Reid for lending us their voice by helping to bring the website alive with audio. Special thanks go to Sally Waldron of World Education for supporting us in bringing this concept to fruition.

Copublished with World Education, Inc.
Published in the United States of America
Manufactured in the United States of America

Printed on acid-free paper

ISBN-13: 978-0-472-03258-7
ISBN-10: 0-472-03258-5

2010   2009   2008   2007   4   3   2   1

Contents

To the Teacher: How to Use This Book

This unique workbook provides a mix of case studies, multimedia, and online work and culminates in project-based activities. It includes a series of units on health care for English language learners who are working in a health care setting or who have friends or relatives in need of support. In each unit, students are presented with a case study of a person with a health issue. After learning about each health issue, students discuss the dilemma posed as they discover ways to help someone in need. The class views videos of professionals sharing their opinions on the case studies. These activities prepare students for an array of projects that offer in-depth exploration of the topics through authentic reading, writing, and speaking tasks. An emphasis is placed on understanding some of the health-related vocabulary useful to communicating with medical personnel. This workbook is accompanied by a companion website at *http://projectcare.worlded.org*.

One thing we want to stress from the outset about the health care information provided in this book: The health information provided is not intended to be exhaustive or comprehensive on any topic, and it can never replace professional advice for individual cases. Please be sure to emphasize this point with students and encourage them to consult a health professional if they or someone they love is ill.

The book can be used in a variety of ways and settings:

- **To supplement** a language skills-based text.

- **To engage students in a topic and in stimulating conversation** before delving into the study of a health care issue using other materials.

- **To augment or to introduce the intensive study of a specific health issue** by moving from medical details of a disease previously covered with a class to a discussion and investigation on how best to help others with the illness.

- **To create small groups of learners that can select an issue of interest** and pursue it as a project-based activity.
- **To integrate technology** into the classroom, mixing face-to-face class time with online reading and projects.

Key Features

There are five main features within each unit:

1. a **preview** (Before You Begin) that introduces students to the health issue and associated vocabulary

2. a **case study and readings on a health issue**

3. a **discussion of the problem posed**

4. **a video clip with input from a professional**

5. **projects** for students to deepen knowledge of an issue and that offer greater opportunity for language practice

Also included are group and writing activities. After projects are shared, students will be asked to evaluate and reflect on how they can implement what they learned into their lives. For more background information on the health topics, see the resources on the companion website: *http://projectcare.worlded.org/resources.html#health.*

Introducing a Unit to Students

Before introducing units to students, we expect that teachers will determine student interest in the topic and get student buy-in, since every student may not be interested in each issue or not currently know someone with each health problem. It is helpful to point out that students will not only improve their English through these activities, but they will gain important knowledge that will be useful in their daily lives, their present work, or in a future career.

We also assume that some general vocabulary words related to health care will be unfamiliar to students. These words do not reflect the reading level of the text. Because these words are fairly basic in the field of health care—commonly used by medical personnel and commonly used by someone describing a health problem—and because they appear frequently throughout the text without glosses, teachers should pre-teach these words before beginning the units. Even if students have some familiarity with these words, it's probably wise to review them:

- addicted/addiction
- diagnose/diagnosis
- disease
- primary care physician
- prognosis
- psychologist
- symptom

For more on the vocabulary that appears in the book, see pages x and xviii.

Before teaching each unit, you should review the material on the companion site *(http://projectcare.worlded.org)* and decide if you will have students focus more on their English in conversation or in writing. Some activities can be done either way with success; only you know what you think would be of greater benefit to your students.

Imagining with Images

By introducing a photo and question as stimuli for discussion, students can activate prior knowledge on the topic and start to emotionally engage with the issues. Students can begin to empathize with a person who has the health problem.

Teaching Ideas

If the class is working on the unit together, you can ask students to share their thoughts about the photo and questions with the whole class. Alternatively, you can give students five minutes to write their answers to the questions, and then ask small groups to talk about them.

Before You Begin

This section taps into learners' prior knowledge and experience with the health topic. The vocabulary presented in **What Vocabulary Do You Already Know?** is directly related to the topic at hand and includes words that will be used throughout the unit. The target health care vocabulary in each unit appears in bold throughout the readings in the unit. Again, these words do <u>not</u> reflect the level of the text, but they do provide basic health care terminology that will be of use to those working in or spending time in a health care setting. The **Your Health Care Dictionary** section at the end of each unit offers a place for students to record the meanings of these important words.

The **What Do You Already Know about the Topic?** activities help students build background knowledge before they seek the answers in the readings that follow.

Teaching Ideas

Although this could be individualized written work, we suggest small groups or pairs because this dynamic often leads to discussion. This can result in interesting interchanges, so we advise checking in with groups to see if they have questions about the material presented.

Previewing the Case Study

The **What You Need to Know** section begins with a short reading that provides students with more information about the health issue. Words and phrases in bold are important to understanding the health issue. General vocabulary that could be challenging appears in color throughout the case study and readings, indicating those words that might be important to preteach or check when reading together with the class.

Teaching Ideas

Learning vocabulary in context, as with any strategy, is sometimes useful depending on the textual clues. Most texts that students will encounter, however, offer very few clues in terms of context (see Folse 2004, *Vocabulary Myths*). Less advanced language learners could have greater difficulty with this approach and might need to consult a dictionary.

Depending on your class's needs, it may be helpful to pre-teach some vocabulary. Your students' level of proficiency in English will also determine how much practice you may have to provide for the words that appear in color. Definitions of these words are provided in each unit after the case study preview (Vocabulary Check). This is because we want students to be able to maximize their understanding of the readings and the health issues. There are a variety of vocabulary development activities you could do with your students to help them learn the words and phrases they do not know. It might be helpful to teach the meanings through class discussion, total physical response (TPR), drawing simple pictures, or analysis of word parts, just to give some examples.

Case Study

If students have not already connected with the health issue, this is where most will. By coming to know "people" with the problem, the case study sets the stage for further reading, reflecting, and investigating. The case study provides information about an individual and the illness and lays out a problem for the person who is trying to help. An attempt was made to include a diverse population throughout the case studies, without any intention of labeling a population as having a propensity toward any particular health issue. If you would like links to more information on the case study approach see *http://projectcare.worlded.org/resources.html#educational*.

Teaching Ideas

The case study can be read in class with the entire class, in small groups, or independently. For example:

1. Ask students to skim the case study, focusing on any subtitles and first and last paragraphs before they read the entire case study silently.

2. You read the case study orally (in part or in its entirety) followed by students reading silently.

3. The case study is read orally as a class with students taking turns reading portions. You can stop and ask questions to check for comprehension and help with pronunciation.

4. The case study can be read at home followed by comprehension questions. Then students are ready to discuss what happens next.

Understanding the Case Study

Questions are designed to ensure that students understand the basic problem of the case study before moving on to consider the consequences of the health issue.

Teaching Ideas

Questions can be answered in writing, for homework, or in class in small groups. Teachers might also use them for an oral comprehension check. Students can also pair up and ask each other questions as conversation practice. Review the answers.

Caring for Someone Who...

Before starting this section, ensure that the class has a good grasp of the issues illustrated in the case studies. The readings that follow the case studies are intended to help formulate a problem for the class to discuss. They end with an implicit question: How can a caregiver help the individual with the illness?

Teaching Ideas

Make sure that students understand that the purpose of this section is to examine the problem posed and think about what advice they might give the caregivers. Most advanced readers will be better able to comprehend this kind of reading if they do so silently.

Increasing Your Understanding: Group Work

The group work activities are an opportunity for students to actively reflect together on the dilemmas posed in the readings. By working together they will not only practice their conversational skills, but they will also learn from each others' experience as they try to apply what they know to a "real-life" situation.

Teaching Ideas

Depending on the activity and the class needs, pairs may be more appropriate than a larger group of three to five students. Visit each group, listening, asking questions, and reinforcing correct answers to the exercises.

Discussion

This section allows learners to begin to engage in constructing their own solutions on how to help before they find out more from their reading, projects, and listening to an expert. Through discussion or writing, students suggest their own ideas on how to help the person with the health issue. Since the **Learning More about the Topic** reading provides additional information on the health issue, teachers might want to consider giving this to students before they start the discussion. This would depend on whether or not you want students to inform their discussion with more background or to use the discussion as a motivation for reading further and learning more about the issue. Either way, as you circulate during the discussion, refer students to the reading particularly when you notice any misconceptions or questions arising.

Learning More about the Topic

After the case study, we provide basic information about the unit's health topic, including information about the larger consequences of not addressing the health issue. As the class works through the remainder of the unit, especially while working on the projects, students will learn more in-depth health information and how to care for someone with the health issue.

Teaching Ideas

Ask the class to read the section silently. Afterward, talk about the information, asking students what information they already knew and what was new for them. Write vocabulary that was troublesome for them on the board. Help with pronunciation and definitions. Answer questions that will help the class suggest solutions to the problem posed in the case study, but point out that their future project work is intended to lead them to investigate more and further build their knowledge on the topic. You can also have student pairs read and discuss the information. Ask student pairs to make two questions about the reading for another student pair to answer. See the health information section at *http://projectcare.worlded.org/resources.html#health* for links to related topics. If students don't have access to the Internet, print out the web pages for them.

Learning More from an Expert

After reading all the material and completing the class discussion regarding what they would do, students should go the appropriate section of the website at *http://projectcare.worlded.org* and click on the video. There, they will hear a professional give an opinion of how to help someone with each health problem.

Teaching Ideas

As an authentic method of assessing comprehension, follow the video by checking listening comprehension just as you might with a reading. You can also ask students to complete listening comprehension quizzes on the website. If necessary, offer to repeat the video. Or ask students to read the transcript, which can be downloaded from the website, while listening to the video a second time. Alternatively, have students read the transcript before viewing the video again.

Afterward, students will discuss questions from the book. There they are asked about their opinion of the expert's advice and what suggestions they now have for the caregiver. They can answer these questions (orally or in writing) in pairs or small groups and then share their answers, or it can be discussed with the whole class. Extend the activity by playing the video again and asking the class to take notes, summarize, or organize it in an outline of steps or suggestions that the expert lists.

Writing

After each video, students are asked to write a paragraph applying what they have learned so far to their own experience or expressing their opinion on aspects of the health situation in the unit.

Teaching Ideas

You may wish to review how to write a well-formed paragraph, such as including a topic sentence, supporting details, and a conclusion. Remind students of pre-writing activities, for example brainstorming in pairs or small groups or creating a mind-map. As an additional pre-writing activity, students can talk together in pairs or small groups, or they can write their responses and discuss them afterwards. In any case, if you plan on having students share their personal experiences, advise them of this ahead of time.

Projects

Each unit contains four projects. We recommend that you use the first project if you plan to have the class work on only one because these projects require the students to use a variety of language skills. Best practice in project-based activity involves assessment, and often teachers use checklists or rubrics so that students and teachers can evaluate student progress. Please see the Project sections of the website for downloadable checklists that you can adapt or go to ***http://projectcare.worlded.org/resources.html# checklists***. Copies are included in the book on pages 114-16.

Teaching Ideas

If you plan to have students choose their projects, review each project introduction and task orally, or ask students to read and decide on two that they prefer. Then, organize students into groups of three or four, according to their interests. When you group students, be sure to consider factors such as students' academic level and experience working in groups. Make sure there is at least one person in each group who has the social and organizational skills to initiate action and facilitate bringing the project to completion. If a group does not include someone like this, it may be difficult for the students to successfully complete the project without a lot of support and guidance from you. If the project is computer-based, it is ideal if one student in the group feels comfortable using computers. This student doesn't necessarily have to know the particular computer program, but he or she should feel comfortable learning it and teaching the others about it. Alternatively, students can group themselves, and then each group can choose which project to work on. Depending on the tasks, the suggested group size is three to four: enough to practice communication but not too many to make it difficult to distribute the responsibilities of the task and make communication challenging. It is also possible to have students work individually if it is more appropriate due to interests, personality, or working style.

While groups are working, walk around, checking in with the groups to make sure they understand the task and to answer questions. We suggest you ask groups to describe their plan. If there is any difference of opinion on what the project entails, help clarify what the project involves. See if students are having difficulty with technology or group interaction. If you see someone working alone, don't be immediately concerned. Check in to see if this is because the group made a plan about distributing the work. Just make sure they plan to share their work at some point to create the final product together.

If it looks like students are having a hard time working as a group, or have individual interests, students can work individually with support from the group. Explain to students that the group work, in and of itself, is important. The process is important, not only the product. This is a good time to show the students the checklist so they understand what you hope they will achieve by this often challenging group work. Make sure to stress to students that the value of working in a group is to practice conversation. If they are advancing to college or work, group work is necessary, and so it's advantageous to learn to work cooperatively. Of course, another advantage of working in a group is tapping each other's knowledge and skills.

Most students are accustomed to writing reports on topics and not investigating a specific question. If students are working on different health issues, encourage them to give a brief overview of the issue, and not an in-depth report, so the audience can contextualize the task and not give so much information that students lose focus on the project task.

You can estimate at least six to eight hours for each project:

- 1 hour to explain the project and organize students into groups, deciding on roles, getting them set up onto computers if necessary

- 2-3 hours on research, including accessing websites and printing them out

- 3 hours completing and executing the project as a group, either in the classroom or as homework

It is best if class time is available for students to work on the project. If projects are not done during class time, students may have difficulties completing the projects. It can be very challenging for students to communicate with each other between class by email or phone, and schedules may not allow then to find time to meet.

Before students begin their work, show them examples of the end product, for example a PowerPoint show or poster. Collect groups' completed work to show to subsequent classes, making sure to get students' permission to share.

Help students balance the time and attention they spend on research with the time and attention on the synthesis of the information and work necessary to complete the project. The teacher should check in to make sure each student has some responsibility and is doing his/her work. It can be difficult for students to address the situation if everyone is not participating and contributing equally.

For projects that require use of technology, it is wise to check ahead that it is working properly. If students need the Internet or software such as PowerPoint, make sure it is installed on the computers and is functioning. The computer lab staff at your school can be a great help here. Ask them to check the computers for you. **It is also important to realize that web links can change at any time, so be sure to check them before the class starts the project.** To find a page that has moved, use the website's internal search or a search engine.

Review how to summarize and not plagiarize the material they research because the tendency for some students when going to a website is to cut and paste information into their own work. Make a schedule for students to submit their work to you to check content, grammar, spelling, sentence structure, and so on. Check and revise students' work periodically, as you normally would do. Take advantage of the fact that students are naturally motivated to do revision before they have to get up to present their project to the class.

Included in the project section of the website are relevant evaluation checklists. Please adapt them according to the objectives of the course and the needs of students. These should be reviewed with the class before beginning work on the projects, so students know what they are responsible for producing. The checklists can be used as is with checkmarks, or you can develop a more robust rubric. To adapt ours or create your own checklist or rubric, see the link provided at *http://projectcare.worlded.org/resources. html#checklists*. Students can evaluate themselves, group members can evaluate each other, or teachers can adapt the checklists to evaluate students. Ask students to use the checklist before they start the project to remind them of their goals and what constitutes a successful project. Encourage students to look at it as a way to stay on track before they're done and to make sure they have done their best.

Ask students to present their work to the class. Presenting the projects is a real motivation for students because they know there is an audience.

For more information about project-based learning see *http://projectcare. worlded.org/resources.html#educational*.

Reflection

Students are asked to write their thoughts on how they improved their language while working on the unit, as well as what they learned about the health topic and caring for others. This can be shared with other students.

Moving On

This section helps students assess what more they need to know about, and how they can apply what they learned in the unit to their lives. This can be shared with classmates.

Your Health Care Dictionary

This section acts like a vocabulary notebook for students. They can easily refer to these pages as they work on the material in the unit or website, and then refer to the words on these pages even after they complete the course. The idea is for students to include whatever information is useful to them to help them remember or understand what the word means. In some cases, this may be a translation. That's okay. You can decide if you want to periodically check student activity on these pages or allow students to come to you if they want to make sure they understand the word/phrase. These pages also include space for students to add other words they want to learn.

Teaching Ideas

If students need some instruction on how to use a dictionary, you can show them how to analyze an entry. Together with the class, find definitions for several words in a unit. Then ask pairs to find several more, and check their work. Alternately, learners can review these words and quiz each other orally, or the teacher can give a written quiz.

What Does It Mean to Be Depressed?

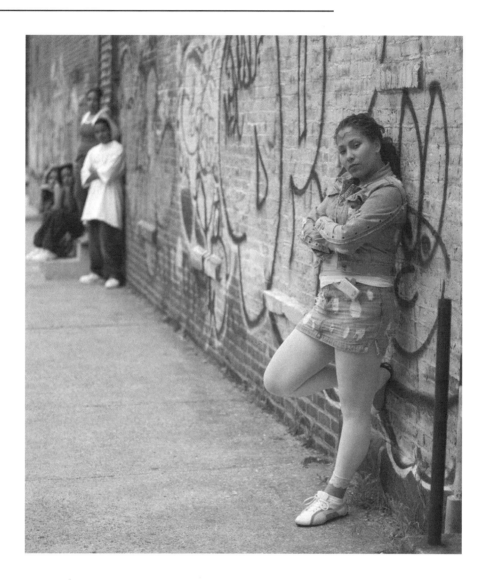

Imagining with Images

What do you think the girl in the photo is feeling? Have you ever felt isolated from others? Have you ever felt alone? Have you known someone who seemed to be sad for a long time?

Before You Begin

What Vocabulary Do You Already Know

Some of the words related to this topic that
or in discussions with health professionals a
words used in this unit. How many do you
plete the unit and learn the meanings of
them to Your Health Care Dictionary pag

anti-depressants	psyc
clinical depression	sui
counseling/counselor	therapy/the...
culture shock	to be/feel down/to be/fee...
hopelessness	to feel numb
insomnia	trigger *(noun and verb)*
mood	

What Do You Already Know about This Topic?

All of us **feel down** at times. **Feeling blue** or sad for a few hours or a few days is normal; it happens to everybody. This general depression or depressed **mood** is not usually a serious health concern. A depressed **mood** that lasts for more than two weeks, however, and does not go away can turn into **clinical depression.**

If someone is depressed, which of these symptoms/behaviors do you think are present?

- ☐ sleeps more hours than the average person
- ☐ sleeps fewer hours than the average person
- ☐ restless and can't sleep
- ☐ cries a lot
- ☐ can't laugh
- ☐ hears imaginary "voices"
- ☐ sees things that aren't there
- ☐ is angry
- ☐ is sad
- ☐ feels tired
- ☐ is often nervous
- ☐ is in pain
- ☐ doesn't feel pain
- ☐ drinks more alcohol than normal
- ☐ eats a lot
- ☐ loses his or her appetite
- ☐ doesn't want to be alone
- ☐ wants to be alone
- ☐ works more than he or she normally does
- ☐ stays at home a lot more than other people
- ☐ wants to only do fun activities
- ☐ doesn't enjoy activities that he or she used to
- ☐ doesn't worry about anything

Now read what the American Academy of Family Physicians says are symptoms of depression. Compare these to what you checked on page 3. Which ones match? Which do not?

- No interest or pleasure in things you used to enjoy
- Feeling sad or empty
- Crying easily or crying for no reason
- Feeling slowed down or feeling restless and unable to sit still
- Feeling worthless or guilty
- Weight gain or loss
- Thoughts about death or **suicide**
- Trouble thinking, recalling things, or focusing on what he or she is doing
- Trouble making everyday decisions
- **Insomnia** or problems sleeping, especially in the early morning, or wanting to sleep all of the time
- Feeling tired all of the time
- Feeling numb emotionally, perhaps even to the point of not being able to cry

1. Answer the following questions. If you feel comfortable and if your teacher asks, talk about your answers with another student.

   - It is normal to feel depressed sometimes. What types of behavior could indicate someone is depressed? When do you know that it's time to seek help from a health professional?

   _____

   _____

   _____

   - Do you know anyone who is depressed? Describe how that person feels and acts.

   _____

   _____

   _____

Previewing the Case Study

What You Need to Know

Preparing to Read the Case Study

Preview the reading about the health topic and the case study. Read about the topic to help you get a better understanding of the vocabulary and issues associated with depression. Important health care-related terms and phrases are in **bold** type. Then read a summary of the case study. Some of the vocabulary words that are in color in the case study are often-used English words that are helpful in many situations. How many of the **bold** or color words/phrases do you already know?

INTERACT ONLINE»

:: Go to *http://projectcare.worlded.org/depression/case.html* to listen to the summary of the case study.

Culture Shock. People who come to live in a new country and culture for the first time usually go through some form of adjustment and often experience **culture shock.** Culture shock has at least four stages:

1. The Honeymoon Stage: "Everything is new and exciting!"

2. The Culture Shock Stage: "Everything is so difficult here!"

3. The Adjustment Stage: "Not everything is quite so bad!"

4. The Acceptance Stage: "Everything may not be perfect here, but I feel at home."

It is typical for people to feel depressed sometime during this process of adjustment. Please describe how you (or someone you know) felt about being part of a new culture and the adjustment process.

_____

_____

_____

_____

SUMMARY OF THE CASE STUDY

Juana Ortiz is a 16-year-old who comes to Chicago to live with her mother Isilma and her sister Rosa in a small apartment. In Venezuela, she used to live in a bigger house. At first, Juana seems to really like her new high school in the United States. Then Juana's behavior changes abruptly. She doesn't seem like herself. Her grades in school suddenly fall, and then she refuses to go to school. Now she rarely goes out with school friends. Juana's mother tries to figure out what is wrong.

Her mother takes Juana to the clinic for a physical exam. The doctor refers her to a therapist. Her mother tries to convince her to go, but Juana refuses. Isilma does not know how she can help Juana.

Vocabulary Check

Definitions of the color words used in the unit follow. Review the definitions to check your understanding of the words and how they are used in the unit.

convince *(verb)* — to cause someone to believe something should be done or is true

divorce *(noun)* — legal ending to a marriage

expressionless *(adjective)* — without emotion or showing one's feeling

figure out *(verb)* — to solve, to understand

hesitant *(adjective)* — unsure

genetic makeup *(noun)* — the combination of genes that define each individual

inherit *(verb)* — to receive something from a parent or relative

isolate *(verb)* — to separate from others, cause to be alone

out of character — not typical, not likely given the person

persuade *(verb)* — to convince or talk someone into or out of something

potentially *(adverb)* — possibly

refer *(verb)* — to direct or guide someone to someone or something else

seem like oneself/herself/himself *(verb)* — appear to be acting the way one usually does

stress/stressors *(noun)* — mental or physical strain or difficulty; events or things that can bring on stress

used to *(verb)* — accustomed to doing or experiencing

Case Study

Juana Ortiz

Juana Ortiz is a 16-year-old youth who came from Venezuela to the United States to live with her mother Isilma and her little sister Rosa. She has been in the United States for six months now. Juana grew up in a large house in a nice area of Caracas. There she attended a private girl's school, until her parents divorced three years ago. Now Juana lives in a small two-bedroom apartment in Chicago, sharing a bedroom with Rosa, her 9-year-old sister. Her plan is to finish high school and then get a job. She secretly dreams of attending university some day.

Symptoms

Juana has not seemed like herself lately. Isilma is concerned because six months ago when Juana started school she used to come home and sit on the living room couch and talk excitedly about her courses, her teachers, and classmates. Now, when she does talk about school, she usually complains about it. Isilma assumes Juana is being a typical teenager. She also realizes that her daughter is now living in a tiny apartment in a different country and attending a new school. Her mother thinks, it must be difficult to speak and listen to English all day.

Isilma is hesitant to talk with Juana's teachers but is concerned and decides to bring a friend to help her translate. Her teachers say that they notice she is not participating in class like in the past months. Her grades are falling. To Isilma, it makes sense that Juana is having difficulty adapting to the U.S. culture and a new school at the same time.

Soon her mother observes other changes in her behavior. Instead of going out with her girlfriends, she spends a lot of time in her room. Juana's sister, Rosa, complains that she never talks to her anymore.

Then one morning, after knocking several times, Isilma enters her room. She can't get Juana out of bed to go to school. Juana pulls the bed covers over her head and yells, "I am not going to school today or ever again!" This behavior is very out of character for Juana; she is normally very polite and respectful. Isilma ignores her behavior and tries talking with her, but she can't find out what's wrong. Juana says she doesn't know what's wrong or how to feel better.

Since then, Juana only gets out of bed to eat and watch TV. She rarely comes out of her room, and if she does, it is at night. Sometimes Isilma gets up in the middle of the night to find her eating junk food and watching movies.

A Diagnosis?

After nagging Juana for a couple of weeks, Isilma is able to persuade Juana to get a physical exam at the neighborhood health clinic. The doctor, however, can't find anything wrong with her physically. The doctor asks her some questions about her eating and sleeping habits, but nothing about school or moving to the United States. He says that her change in sleeping and eating habits and her lack of interest in things she used to enjoy can be signs of depression. Juana listens quietly. Her face remains expressionless while the doctor suggests that she see a **psychologist** or **therapist.** After they leave the building, Juana is angry. She yells and says she is not crazy. Isilma tells her that she doesn't think that she is crazy, but she still tells her that she has to go to the appointment. They walk the rest of the way home in silence.

Understanding the Case Study

Answer each question about the case study. Use complete sentences.

1. Describe the changes in Juana's life.

   _____

   _____

2. What symptoms of depression can you find in Juana's behavior?

   _____

   _____

3. Did Juana just wake up one day and decide she didn't want to go to school, or did her unhappiness occur gradually? How do you know?

   _____

   _____

4. What stage of culture shock is Juana in? Explain.

   _____

   _____

5. What was Juana's reaction to going to see a psychologist or therapist?

   _____

   _____

6. Will Juana go to the appointment? Why or why not?

   _____

   _____

Caring for Someone Who Is Depressed

Each time Isilma goes to Juana's bedroom door to tell her to get ready for an appointment with the **therapist,** Juana refuses to go. After a few times, her mother gives up and stops making appointments. Juana doesn't want to talk to anyone about how she feels. Isilma hopes that her sadness and feelings of **hopelessness** will pass. She tries to figure out what caused Juana to change.

Isilma asks her friends and relatives for advice. Some relatives agree that the cause might be all the changes in Juana's life. A man who lives upstairs thinks Juana is lazy and needs structure in her life, such as getting a part-time job. Others say they think **feeling down** is common for teenagers, and it is just a stage of growing up.

At first, Isilma thinks that she is helping Juana by letting her take a little time off from school to get used to being in a new culture. But soon Isilma becomes frustrated, and eventually she goes to the library to find a book or to get more information on the Internet.

It quickly becomes clear to Isilma that Juana is depressed and that it could be caused by **culture shock.** What Isilma really needs to know is how she can help her daughter, especially if she can't convince Juana to go to a **therapist** or for **counseling.**

Increasing Your Understanding

Group Work

1. Complete the chart. Work with a partner. In the first column, describe what you know about Juana's life in Venezuela. In the second column, describe what you know about Juana's life in the U.S. Try to remember what you read, or go back and re-read the reading for information.

Juana's Life in VENEZUELA	Juana's Life in THE UNITED STATES

2. Compare the diagram. Work with a partner. Juana is depressed. Her depression affects her life and creates problems for her and her family. What are some of these problems? Review the case study for ideas. Add more circles if you need to.

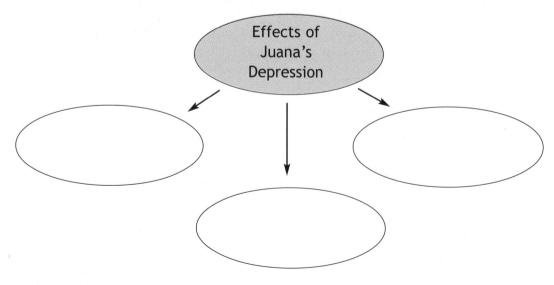

Discussion—What Should Isilma Do?

Discuss the questions in a small group. Try to use some of these phrases.

Phrases Used to Agree	Phrases Used to Disagree
I agree.	Sorry, but I disagree.
I see it the same as you do.	I see it differently.
I can live with that.	I really don't think it's a good idea to....
It seems like a good idea.	
That has been my experience.	I don't think....
I can't say I disagree with....	That hasn't been my experience.
That sounds (about) right to me.	If are you asking my opinion, I....
Your point is well taken.	That might be true, but....
	I see your point, but....

1. What do you think caused Juana's depression? Will that affect the kind of advice you give to Isilma?

2. Do you think Juana's depression is serious or not? Does she have **clinical depression**? Why or why not?

3. What do you think are the best ways Isilma can help her daughter?

Learning More about the Topic*

Depression affects men, women, and children. If left untreated, it can last for months, years, or a lifetime. It can affect a person's thoughts, feelings, overall health, and a person's ability to work and enjoy life. Some experts estimate that 10 to 20 percent of the people working today in the United States are **clinically depressed.**

Sometimes depression appears in several members of a family. These people may **inherit** a **genetic makeup** that makes it more likely to become depressed. However, it is often the case that an event **triggers** sadness or a feeling of **hopelessness,** and that feeling doesn't go away. This can sometimes be what is called situational depression. According to the American Academy of Family Physicians, depression that lasts for two or more weeks can become **clinical depression.** Events that **trigger** depression include:

- The loss of someone or something important such as the death of a loved one, a divorce, the loss of a job, breaking up with a long-time partner, or losing a friend or pet.

- Physical changes in the body that are potentially life-changing like cancer and heart attacks.

- The **stress** or **stressors** of a major life event such as moving to an unfamiliar place (new country, new city) that makes someone feel isolated or lonely.

- A combination of these events or more than one type of loss over a short period of time.

Whether a person suffers from situational or **clinical depression,** the main symptoms are:

- a depressed **mood** most of the day, nearly every day

- a loss of interest or pleasure in all or most activities

Although depression is a real illness, many people never seek help for it because they don't realize it is an illness. They are ashamed to talk about it, or they hope to "snap out of it." But getting help can stop the depression. Those who don't get help can cause themselves and

---

*Although the information in this book might be helpful, it does not replace professional advice for individual cases. You should consult a health professional if you or a loved one has a serious illness.

others to suffer with the effects of depression much longer than they have to. For example, it can lead to physical illness or problems with family, work, or school.

Health care professionals today are especially concerned about young and old people who are depressed and may try to **commit suicide**. According to the Centers for Disease Control and Prevention, **suicide** is the second leading cause of death for college-age students (ages 18-23). **Suicide** rates increase with age and are very high among those 65 years and older. Older adults who are suicidal are more likely to have physical illnesses or to be divorced or widowed.

Fortunately there are many things you can do for depression. If you are depressed for two weeks or longer, you should talk with your doctor and see if the cause is due to a physical condition.

Two of the most common treatments often used together to relieve depression are:

1. talking to a mental health professional (**psychiatrist**, **psychologist**, social worker, mental health **counselor**)
2. taking **anti-depressants** over a period of time

For some people, a stay in a hospital can give them careful supervision, intensive treatment, and a sense of security and safety while being treated.

In addition, there are some other things people can do to help themselves:

- Talk to family members, friends, or community leaders (such as church leaders, teachers, and family doctors).
- Stay healthy by getting enough sleep, exercising, and eating well.
- Avoid alcohol and other recreational drugs.
- Do things that make you feel better such as hobbies, spending time with friends.
- Meditate, pray, or do relaxation techniques.

Learning More from an Expert: Video

INTERACT ONLINE»

:: Go to *http://projectcare.worlded.org/depression/video.html* to watch a video about culture shock and depression. You will hear a professional giving an opinion about what Isilma can do to help Juana. Before you watch you might want to review some vocabulary used in the video at *http://projectcare.worlded.org/depression/vocab.html*. After you complete the listening activity, do the activity below as part of a group or independently.

Discuss/Write

1. Do you agree with the expert's advice? Why or why not?

2. Considering what you have learned so far in this unit, what do you think are the most important steps Isilma should take?

Writing

Give your opinion by answering each question in a well-developed paragraph.

1. Is depression a problem in your culture/home country? What would a family in your home culture/country do to help someone who might be depressed?

_____

_____

_____

_____

_____

_____

_____

_____

_____

_____

_____

_____

_____

_____

_____

_____

_____

_____

2. Did you ever experience culture shock? Did it make you feel depressed? What helped you?

_____

_____

_____

_____

_____

_____

_____

_____

_____

_____

_____

_____

_____

_____

_____

_____

_____

_____

_____

_____

_____

Projects

One in eight teenagers becomes clinically depressed. Learn what you can about depression and how you can help others who suffer from it. The projects will help improve your English conversation, writing, and reading skills and help you prepare yourself and your classmates to support someone with depression.

INTERACT ONLINE»

:: The following projects were designed so that you can go to the Internet and other resources to find more information about depression and how to care for people who have it. You and your teacher may use a checklist to evaluate your work. To find updated links to health information and checklists that will help you with your projects, go to the Project Care website at *http://projectcare.worlded.org/depression/projects.html.*

Project #1—Role Play

Introduction

Isilma tried hard to help Juana. If she had more knowledge about depression, how could she have helped Juana more? Could Juana's teachers and friends have helped?

Task

Your task is to write and perform a role play of Juana's interactions with other people. Include conversations and nonverbal behaviors (posture, facial expressions, ways people move, etc.). Show helpful as well as unhelpful ways to interact with Juana.

Skills

Critical thinking, research, writing, acting, working in a group, making a presentation

Process

1. Make sure you read and understand the instructions before you begin working on your project.
2. Discuss the following in a group: Does anyone in the group know someone with depression or want to share his or her experience with it? Does anyone have training or work experience with people who have depression? Share knowledge with the group.
3. Go to the Project Care website *(http://projectcare.worlded.org/depression/information.html#project1)*. You will find helpful information that you can use in your project.
4. Review the case study and pay special attention to the interactions Juana had with people.
5. Discuss Juana's interactions with her family and friends. Did they help her? Were there better ways to help her?
6. Decide which role(s) each student will play:
    a. Juana
    b. Juana's mother Isilma
    c. Her sister Rosa
    d. Juana's doctor
7. Discuss how to write the script. Then write the script, making sure each person has equal opportunity to speak in the drama. It does not have to be a complete drama; each role can be in a separate scene.
8. Make questions to ask the class before the role play. The questions should help classmates think about interactions between Juana and others. For example: Which conversations were helpful? Which were not helpful? Why? What would be better ways to handle the situation?
9. Give your work to the teacher to check so you can revise it if necessary.

10. Practice so that you don't have to read from the script.
11. Set up the classroom for the role play. Write the questions for the class on the board. Have the class sit in a circle with a space in the middle for the group to perform the role play. Present the role play.
12. With the class, have a discussion on the best way to help people who are depressed by asking the class to respond to the questions on the board.

Project #2—Make a Song or Music Video

Introduction
Many people have misunderstandings of what depression is. They do not understand causes, effects, and treatments for depression. What important information should people know about depression so they can help friends and family?

Task
Your task is to write a song or make a simple music video to teach important information people should know about depression so they can help. You can also educate people on what it feels like to be depressed.

Skills
Critical thinking, research, writing, acting, producing a video, working in a group, performing

Process
1. Review the case study.
2. Discuss the following in a group: Does anyone in the group know someone with depression? Does anyone have training or work experience with people who have depression? Share knowledge with the group.
3. Go to the Project Care website *(http://projectcare.worlded.org/depression/ information.html#project2)*. You will find helpful information that you can use in your project.
4. Read newspaper and magazine articles or books to find out more experts' advice and information on living with depression, its causes, symptoms, and treatments.
5. Learn the basics of how to write a song. Go to the Project Care website *(http://projectcare.worlded.org/depression/information.html#project2)*. You will find helpful information that you can use in your project. Record the song on a tape recorder, computer, or video camera. You can also try creating a simple music video.
6. Decide how your group will share the work:
   a. Writer for the lyrics
   b. Writer for the music (or choose an existing song to use for the music)
   c. Musicians (if performing your own music)
   d. Director (for music video)
   d. Actors/actresses and/or artists (for music video)
   e. Editor (for music video)
7. Practice your performance (and film, if making video).
8. Have your teacher view a practice performance to check it so you can revise it if necessary.
9. Present your song or music video to the class.

Project #3—Interview

Introduction
To understand depression, it helps to talk with someone who has experienced it. What can you learn about depression from interviewing someone who has it or who had it earlier?

Task
Interview someone who has had depression. Present what you learned to the class.

Skills
Listening, forming questions, interviewing, research, critical thinking, working in a group, making a presentation

Process
1. Review the case study.
2. Discuss the following in a group: Does anyone in the group know someone with depression? Does anyone have training or work experience with people who have depression? Share knowledge with the group.
3. Go to the Project Care website *(http://projectcare.worlded.org/depression/ information.html#project3)*. You will find helpful information that you can use in your project.
4. Think of questions to ask someone who has depression. Think of questions to help you understand how the person thinks and feels. For example: What were signs of your depression that family and friends did and didn't recognize? What did family and friends do that helped you the most? Each group member makes at least two questions.
5. Find someone with depression who is comfortable being interviewed. If your group doesn't know someone to interview, you can try contacting an advocacy/educational organization. Use an Internet search engine such as Google™ and search for "mental health state resources guide." Click on your state to find advocacy organizations to contact. If you have difficulty, ask health care professionals if they would talk about their experience helping others who suffer from depression. If you need help, ask your teacher.
6. Ask the interviewee if she or he prefers to be interviewed in class or outside of class. Alternatively, each student in the group can interview a different person. If the group will interview one person together, each group member asks at least two questions. If you will interview outside of class, take notes on the interviewee's answers.
7. Prepare a presentation on what your group learned from the interview about what it's like to live with depression. Each group member is responsible for an equal part of the presentation.
8. Give your work to the teacher to check, so that you can revise it if necessary.
9. Present to the class.

Project #4—Depression at Different Ages

Introduction
Symptoms and treatment for depression in youth, adults, and the elderly have similarities and differences. What are they?

Task
Your task is to research the differences and similarities in symptoms and treatments for depression among youth, adults, and the elderly. Make a web page or brochure to share your findings with the class.

Skills
Critical thinking, research, making a web page/making a brochure, working in a group, making a presentation

Process
1. Review the case study.
2. Discuss the following in a group: Does anyone in the group know someone with depression? Does anyone have training or work experience with people who have depression? Share knowledge with the group.
3. Group members list similarities and differences they think exist in symptoms and treatment for depression among youth, adults, and the elderly.
4. Go to the Project Care website *(http://projectcare.worlded.org/depression/ information.html#project4)*. You will find helpful information that you can use in your project. Go to the library and talk to professionals to learn more.
5. Look at your group list and add or delete, based on what you learned.
6. Choose one similarity or difference that is important for people to know. As an alternative, different presentations can be created for each age.
7. Write about the information on the similarity or difference you researched.
8. Meet in groups and read each others' writing. Give feedback to each other— what do you like? What is clear? What is confusing? Students edit their writing and make a final version.
9. Make the web page using a free template on the Internet. Each group member puts his or her information on the website. To make the brochure, you can use the Microsoft Word template.
10. Give your work to the teacher to check, so that you can revise it if necessary.
11. Present your information on the web page for the class.

Reflection

Review the activities in this unit, and then evaluate your progress by answering the questions.

What did you learn about...

- **English**—How did you improve in the areas of reading, writing, speaking, or listening? List at least two new words or grammar points that you learned.

_____

_____

_____

_____

- **Health**—What did you learn about depression or the health field in general? List at least two new things you learned.

_____

_____

_____

_____

- **Caregiving**—What did you learn about how you can help others? List at least two new things you learned about how you can help a person with depression.

_____

_____

_____

_____

Moving On

What do you need or want to learn more about?

_____

_____

_____

_____

_____

Can you think of ways that you can apply what you learned in this unit to your life or job?

_____

_____

_____

_____

_____

Your Health Care Dictionary

List the vocabulary words and expressions you learned that are related to health care. Write a definition or synonym next to each. Then write a sentence that uses the word. An example has been done for you.

1. counseling

   help or advice from a therapist or specialist

   To help her understand her depression, she decided to go to counseling.

2. _____

   _____

   _____

3. _____

   _____

   _____

4. _____

   _____

   _____

5. _____

   _____

   _____

6. _____

   _____

   _____

7.

_____

_____

8.

_____

_____

9.

_____

_____

10.

_____

_____

11.

_____

_____

12.

_____

_____

13.

_____

_____

14.

_____

_____

15.

_____

_____

16.

_____

_____

17.

_____

_____

18.

_____

_____

What Is the Difference between Alcoholism and Alcohol Abuse?

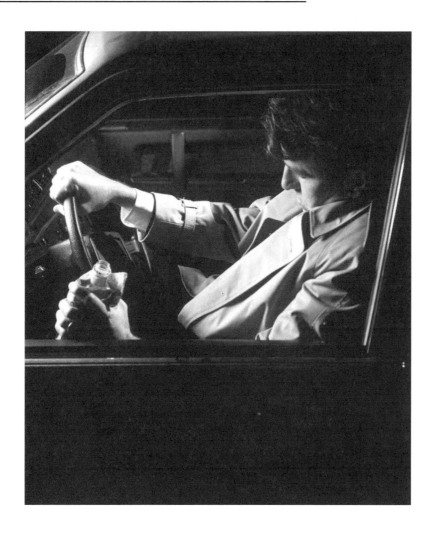

Imagining with Images

Imagine you are walking by your neighbor's house one evening and you see him drive his car into the trash bins next to the driveway. When you go over to talk to him to see if he's okay, you notice he has an open liquor bottle. Should you say or do anything? Do you think this event could mean he is an alcoholic? How do you know?

Before You Begin

What Vocabulary Do You Already Know?

Some of the words related to this topic that you may hear in your work or in discussions with health professionals are listed. You will find these words used in the unit. How many do you already know? As you complete the unit and learn the meanings of these words and phrases, add them to Your Health Care Dictionary pages at the end of the unit.

alcohol dependence

addiction

consumption limits

hangover

sober/sobriety

substance abuse/alcohol abuse

[to be/to drive] under the influence

withdrawal symptoms

What Do You Already Know about This Topic?

Doctors and health professionals sometimes use the expression unhealthy alcohol use to describe a range of behavior that describes a problem with alcohol. Some people's behavior could indicate possible alcohol abuse or dependence, while others might just be beginning to have a problem.

1. Work with a small group to complete the questions based on what you already know about unhealthy alcohol use.

   1. Men who have more than _____drink(s) a week might have a problem.

   2. Men who have more than _____drink(s) on each occasion might have a problem.

   3. People over age 65 and women who have more than _____ drink(s) a week might have a problem.

   4. People over age 65 and women who have more than _____ drink(s) on each occasion might have a problem.

2. Check your answers against the information given in the reading on page 33. What surprises you about the correct answers?

Definitions of Unhealthy Alcohol Use

What is unhealthy alcohol use? The term unhealthy alcohol use refers to a variety of behaviors described as at-risk drinking to **alcohol dependence** (National Institute of Alcohol Abuse and Alcoholism [NIAAA] website 2007). Drinking that is becoming "at-risk" means that the person is drinking more than the limits that are safe. The person is therefore likely to suffer illness, injury, or social/legal problems as a result of the alcohol.

The recommended **consumption limits** according to NIAAA are two standard drinks per drinking occasion or 14 standard drinks per week for men and one standard drink per drinking occasion or seven drinks per week for women or anyone over the age of 65. A standard drink is defined as 12 grams of pure alcohol, the amount contained in about 12 ounces of beer, 5 ounces of wine, or 1.5 ounces of distilled spirits.

Once someone experiences a harmful event that is a direct result of consuming alcohol like an injury, illness, or social/legal problem (such as poor grades, an argument with parents, or a driving **under the influence** violation), he or she is considered to be a harmful drinker.

At the extreme of at-risk/harmful drinking is **alcohol abuse** and **alcohol dependence** as defined by criteria established in the American Psychiatric Association's *Diagnostic and Statistical Manual of Mental Disorders, Fourth Edition* (DSM-IV).

3. Answer the following questions. If you feel comfortable and if your teacher asks, talk about your answers with another student.

   - Many people drink alcohol without having any problems. At what point do you think drinking alcohol becomes a problem?

   _____

   _____

   - In your opinion, is someone who gets drunk every weekend an alcoholic? Explain why or why not.

   _____

   _____

- List any symptoms of alcoholism that you know.

_____

_____

- Do you know anyone (neighbor, classmate, friend, etc.) who has this problem? Are there people in the person's life who are trying to help? Are they able to help? How can you tell?

_____

_____

Previewing the Case Study

What You Need to Know

Preparing to Read the Case Study

Preview the reading about the health topic and the case study. Read about the topic to help you get a better understanding of the vocabulary and issues associated with alcoholism. Important health care-related terms and phrases are in **bold** type. Then read a summary of the case study. Some of the vocabulary words that are in color in the case study are often-used English words that are helpful in many situations. How many of the **bold** or color words/phrases do you already know?

INTERACT ONLINE»
:: Go to *http://projectcare.worlded.org/alcoholism/vocab.html* to listen to the summary of the case study.

What Is Alcoholism? According to the NIAAA (2007), alcoholism or **alcohol dependence** is a disease where the need for alcohol in the body is so strong that the person cannot function without it.

What Is Alcohol Abuse? Alcohol abuse is different from alcoholism. It is sometimes called "problem drinking." People who are abusing alcohol do not have an extreme craving for alcohol, a loss of control over how much they drink, or physical dependence on alcohol.

SUMMARY OF THE CASE STUDY

Takashi Sato's wife, Amy, is concerned about the severity of her husband's drinking problem. He has been drinking a lot over the past year and is now coming home every night of the week **under the influence.** She is very worried about him, and she has no friend or relative to turn to for help. Feeling that she is at the end of her rope, she decides to send an email to a medical website to seek advice. She explains how her husband is **sober** during the day but is getting drunk every weeknight. She is afraid to keep telling him that she thinks he is drinking too much, but Amy wants him to alter his behavior.

Vocabulary Check

Definitions of the color words used in the unit follow. Review the definitions to check your understanding of the words and how they are used in the unit.

accuse *(verb)* — to blame someone

alter *(verb)* — to change

at the end of her rope *(idiom)* — to feel like there is nothing else to try to help a situation

bring up *(verb)* — to raise

cover *(verb)* [as in health insurance]— to pay the costs of

customary *(adjective)* — common or expected

defensive *(adjective)* — protective of oneself

lab tech(nician) *(noun)* — someone who works in a medical laboratory

seek [advice] *(verb)* — to request help

severity *(adverb)* — strength or seriousness

stumble *(verb)* — to have trouble walking

turn to *(verb)* — to depend on, ask for help from

Case Study

Takashi Sato

Takashi is a 34-year-old medical lab technician who met his wife after he came to the United States from Japan. Amy was born in the United States. Her family is originally from Italy. They have a 13-year-old child, Akira, and live just outside Seattle, Washington. Amy is worried that Takashi has a serious problem with alcohol.

Symptoms

Takashi's drinking has gotten worse over the last two years. Amy feels that she is at the end of her rope, and she doesn't know who to turn to for help. Amy has no close friends and doesn't have any relatives she feels comfortable talking to about this situation. No one in her family has ever had a problem with alcohol. She decides to go to the Internet for information and support. She knows that she can send a message about a problem and get suggestions from others, and none of her family members will know about it. This is a copy of the email she sent. The doctor's response follows.

Dear Doctor Thomas,

I'm really happy that my Japanese husband has found some Japanese co-workers here in the United States, but since he met them, he's been drinking a lot. He meets them every evening after work, and they get drunk. Then he drives home and stumbles into the house, singing at the top of his lungs, which wakes up our teen-aged son. I'm worried about the effect that Takashi's behavior is having on our son. If it scares me, it must really scare Akira.

I think that my husband may already have a serious drinking problem. I know that in Japan this kind of after-work drinking is quite common, but now he lives in America. Do you think he is doing this because it is customary in Japan? Even if it is a custom in Japan, how can I get him to stop?

I'm afraid that he will get angry if I am always telling him to stop, so I don't. I love my husband. He's a good father, and he works hard for our family. I hope you can tell me what I can do to help him.

Yours truly,
Anxious Amy

––––––––––––––

A Diagnosis?

Dear Amy,

Your husband sounds like a good man. It is true that many Japanese men (in Japan) go out to bars after work to relax and build stronger relationships with co-workers. This custom by itself does not make him an alcoholic. But without talking with your husband, I can't make a diagnosis. However, he does have a problem with his drinking. I say this because I am particularly worried about his **driving** while **under the influence.** In addition, your concern about how his behavior could be harmful to your son is already affecting your marriage.

When your husband is **sober,** I strongly suggest you speak with him about your concerns. Try to clearly tell him how you feel when he comes home drunk and your fears about how it will affect your son. Once he knows how upsetting it is for you and your child, he might realize the severity of his problem and alter his behavior. If he can do that, then this is probably not alcoholism. In any case, I believe all of you, including your son, will need support. I suggest you talk to a counselor in your area. This person can advise you and give you names of groups and organizations that can help you and your family.

Understanding the Case Study

Answer each question about the case study. Use complete sentences.

1. Why is Amy worried?

2. Why does Amy send an email about this problem?

3. What advice does Amy get?

4. What are some emotions Amy is feeling?

5. What bothers Amy the most about Takashi's drinking?

6. Why doesn't Amy want to tell Takashi to stop drinking?

7. Does the doctor say that Takashi is an alcoholic? Why or why not?

_____

_____

8. Do you think Amy was satisfied with the doctor's answer? Why or why not?

_____

_____

9. What do you think Amy will do next?

_____

_____

Caring for Someone
Who Drinks a Lot

One Saturday morning at breakfast when Takashi is recovering from a **hangover,** Amy asks, "Don't you think you are drinking too much?" Takashi becomes angry and defensive when he answers Amy: "I just like to go out with my friends and relax. I work hard, you know. And maybe you are the one with a problem. You have to have a glass of wine with dinner every night. At least I don't drink on the weekends."

Amy doesn't say anything more. She decides to wait for the upcoming vacation, when they are both relaxed, to bring up the topic again. This time she tries not to accuse him but to talk about her feelings. She explains how his drinking upsets her. At first, Takashi defends himself by saying, "I can stop anytime." When she explains her fears about him drinking and driving, he promises that he will take a bus home if he has had a lot to drink. When Amy begins to cry, Takashi complains that going out after work and drinking with co-workers is a custom in Japan and is important for his career.

After their talk, though, Amy is hopeful, but she is still worried that he has a drinking problem and may even be **addicted** to alcohol.

After their vacation, Takashi seems to be trying to change. The first two nights he comes home from work and does not go out with his co-workers. However, he starts smoking again (something he hadn't done since he moved to the United States) and at night sits quietly watching TV with Amy and Akira. The next evening, though, Takashi arrives home late and has beer on his breath. The week ends with Takashi's car screeching into the driveway at midnight.

Amy now realizes that she can't make her husband stop drinking, but she is upset about his broken promises to stop drinking, which is affecting their marriage. Amy feels that she can't live with this situation the way it is, but she doesn't know what to else to do.

Amy thought about Dr. Thomas's advice, but their health insurance covers her for only a few visits to a counselor. She has heard people talk about treatment or rehabilitation centers, where people with **substance abuse** problems go to get help. Amy, however, does not want others to know about her family's problem. "I know that I am not the only one who has this problem, but I still feel so alone," Amy thinks. That night, she pours an extra glass of wine for herself.

Increasing Your Understanding

Group Work

Complete the chart. Work with a partner. In the first column, list things that seem to make Takashi continue to drink beyond his limit. In the second column, write things that might help Takashi stop drinking. Try to remember what you read, or go back and re-read the case study for information.

Things that might make Takashi continue drinking beyond his limit	Things that might help Takashi to stop or cut back on his drinking

Discussion—What Should Amy Do?

1. Does Takashi have a drinking problem that he can stop? If so how?

2. Do you think he is an alcoholic? Why or why not?

3. Is it possible for Amy to get Takashi to stop drinking? If so, how? If not, what should she do next?

4. What can Amy do to help her son understand Takashi's behavior and about responsible use of alcohol?

5. Do you think Amy has a problem with alcohol?

Learning More about the Topic*

Alcoholism, also known as **alcohol dependence**, is a disease that includes four symptoms:

- *craving*—a strong need, or urge, to drink
- *loss of control*—not being able to stop drinking once drinking has begun
- *physical dependence*—**withdrawal symptoms**, such as nausea, sweating, shakiness, and anxiety after stopping drinking
- *tolerance*—the need to drink more alcohol to feel its effects

Although treatment for alcoholism is possible, a person with a history of alcoholism (or drinking problem) has high risk for a relapse. Some experts believe that individuals with a history of alcoholism cannot begin drinking again without the problem returning and that it is not possible for an alcoholic to drink any type of alcohol and remain healthy.

Alcohol abuse is different from alcoholism. Because there is no physical dependency, alcohol abuse can be easier to treat. **Alcohol abuse** is when a person drinks and has one of the following results from drinking during a one-year period:

- not fulfilling work, school, or home responsibilities
- engaging in dangerous situations, such as drinking while driving
- legal problems related to drinking, such as going to jail for driving drunk
- problems with relationships caused by drinking or that get worse because of it

Alcoholism is different from **alcohol abuse**, but the effects can also be experienced by someone who is suffering from alcoholism.

One of the most important issues surrounding **alcohol abuse** and alcoholism is **driving** drunk or **under the influence (DUI)**. The National Institute of Alcohol Abuse and Alcoholism estimates that 39 percent of all

*Although the information in this book might be helpful, it does not replace professional advice for individual cases. You should consult a health professional if you or a loved one has a serious illness.

traffic deaths in 2004 in the United States were the result of the driver or drivers being **"under the influence."** There is roughly one traffic death due to alcohol every 31 minutes in the U.S. "Driving while intoxicated" (DWI) is also a police/legal term for **driving under the influence**. If police suspect a driver has been drinking, the driver will probably be pulled over, tested, charged, and sometimes jailed.

Binge drinking is a phrase often used to refer to another type of problem drinking. This occurs when someone goes days without alcohol but then decides to drink four or five drinks in one sitting. This can cause the individual to vomit, to lose consciousness, and to lose memories (that is, to have blackouts). This can also have severe health consequences such as dehydration of the body, high blood alcohol level, heart failure, and stroke, which can cause death in extreme cases.

In the United States there are many national and local resources available to help someone who may have a drinking problem. There are also some that exist to help friends and families of a person with a drinking problem. These include Alcoholics Anonymous, Al-anon, and other 12-step programs. Of course, medical doctors are also a good place to start. Investigate some sources of help in your local community for someone with a drinking problem.

Learning More from an Expert: Video

INTERACT ONLINE»

:: Go to *http://projectcare.worlded.org/alcoholism/video.html* to watch a video about alcohol abuse and alcoholism. You will hear a professional giving an opinion about what Amy can do to help her family. Before you watch you might want to review some vocabulary used in the video at *http://projectcare.worlded.org/alcoholism/vocab.html*. After you complete the listening activity, do the activity below as part of a group or independently.

Discuss/Write

1. Do you agree with the expert's advice? Why or why not?

2. Considering what you have learned so far in this unit, what do you think are the most important steps Amy should take?

Writing

Give your opinion by answering each question in a well-developed paragraph.

1. Is alcoholism or alcohol abuse a problem in your culture/home country? How do you know?

_____

_____

_____

_____

_____

_____

_____

_____

_____

_____

_____

_____

_____

_____

_____

_____

_____

2. What would you do if your friend or family member had a drinking problem and you thought that he or she might be an alcoholic? Be specific.

_____

_____

_____

_____

_____

_____

_____

_____

_____

_____

_____

_____

_____

_____

_____

_____

_____

_____

Projects

Every year, companies that sell alcohol spend more on advertising and trying to get people to use alcohol than companies selling any other product. More than 100,000 people die in the United States from alcohol abuse each year by driving drunk, diseases of the liver, falls, and other indirect effects. By learning more about alcoholism and alcohol abuse you can prepare yourself and your classmates to help those who suffer from it. The projects will help improve your English conversation, writing, and reading skills and help you prepare yourself and your classmates to support someone who has a problem with alcohol.

INTERACT ONLINE»

:: The following projects were designed so that you can go to the Internet and other resources to find more information about alcoholism and alcohol abuse and how to care for people who have these problems. You and your teacher may use a checklist to evaluate your work. To find updated links to health information and checklists that will help you with your projects, go to the Project Care website at *http:// project care.worlded.org/alcoholism/projects.html*.

Project #1—What Is It Like for the Child? Akira's Perspective

Introduction
Growing up in a family where someone has a problem with alcohol abuse can be very difficult. What are the possible academic and social effects? Are there other effects? What are the chances that children will develop a problem with alcohol?

Task
Make a PowerPoint presentation or a poster(s) to show the possible effects alcoholism has on children academically, socially, and in other ways, and the chances that children will develop the same problem.

Skills
Critical thinking, research, writing, presenting, working in groups, making a PowerPoint presentation

Process
1. Make sure you read and understand the instructions before you begin working on your project.
2. Review the case study, and discuss how you think Akira's life was affected by Takashi's drinking.
3. Discuss the following in a group: Does anyone in the group know someone who is an alcoholic? Does anyone have training or work experience with people who are alcoholics? Share knowledge with the group.
4. Choose different resources to research the effects on children of living in a family where alcohol abuse is present.
5. Go to the Project Care website *(http://projectcare.worlded.org/alcoholism/information.html#project1)*. You will find helpful information that you can use in your project.
6. Visit an open meeting of Adult Children of Alcoholics.
7. Group members discuss information you learned. Decide what information from each person's research to include in the presentation.
8. Make a PowerPoint slide with the information the group decided to include from his or her research.
9. Make a list of questions to ask the class. For example, you can ask others to share their own knowledge, experiences, and opinions. You might ask for ideas on how to help children in this situation.
10. Give your work to the teacher to check so that you can revise it if necessary.
11. Present the PowerPoint slide show to the class.
12. As a group, ask the class the questions you prepared.

Project #2—What Help Is Available in Your Area?

Introduction
Amy did not think that she could talk about this problem with her friends or family, and she didn't consider counseling because she didn't think she could afford to pay for it. What resources are available in your community for people with problems related to alcohol or any substance abuse problem? Are there any that are free or low-cost?

Task
Your task is to make a spreadsheet with information about resources available in your area for people with problems related to alcohol or any other kind of substance abuse.

Skills
Critical thinking, research, creating charts or tables in spreadsheets or word processing, working in a group, making presentations

Process
1. Review the case study.
2. Discuss the following in a group: Does anyone in the group know someone who is an alcoholic? Does anyone have training or work experience with people who are alcoholics? Share knowledge with the group.
3. Go to the Project Care website *(http://projectcare.worlded.org/alcoholism/ information.html#project2)*.
4. List the resources available for adults, for teenagers, and for children in school.
   a. List some ways to find out more about each kind of support.
   b. Ask classmates, friends, or family who work in the field of alcohol abuse.
   c. Use an Internet search engine. Type something like: **find help alcoholism**.
   d. Check with your school's counselor.
   e. Look in the phone book's yellow pages. Try looking under **alcohol abuse and addiction treatment**.
   f. Check with the department of public health in your city.
5. Choose which resources to use. Divide the resources among the group members.
6. Put the information the group finds about resources in a chart using a spreadsheet program, such as Excel, or create tables in Word.
7. Give your work to the teacher to check so that you can revise it if necessary.
8. Distribute copies to the class and others in the community.

Project #3—The Rest of the Story

Introduction

At some point or another, many families have to deal with alcohol-related health issues. How the family deals with the issue depends on the situation and the choices of the family members. What is one possible happy ending for Amy's family? What is one possible unhappy ending?

Task

Your task is to continue Amy's story in two different ways. Write one happy ending and one unhappy ending.

Skills

Critical thinking, research, writing, working in a group, making presentations

Process

1. Review the case study.
2. Discuss the following in a group: Does anyone in the group know someone who is abusing alcohol or fighting alcoholism? Does anyone have training or work experience with people who have drinking problems? Share knowledge with the group.
3. Learn more about alcohol abuse and alcoholism.
4. Go to the Project Care website *(http://projectcare.worlded.org/alcoholism/ information.html#project3)*. You will find helpful information that you can use in your project.
5. Find newspaper or magazine articles or books at your local library.
6. Divide the group so that half the students are working on writing a draft of the story with the happy ending and half the students are working on writing a draft of the story with the unhappy ending. Make sure to include aspects of the family's situation, conflicts between the family members, and choices they make that could lead to the ending. Don't forget to add what people did to improve the situation or make it worse.
7. Students in the group should meet in pairs and read each other's drafts. Give feedback to each other—what do you like? What is clear? What is confusing? Students edit their stories and make a final version.
8. Practice reading out loud. Make copies for the students and teacher.
9. Make a list of discussion questions to ask the class. Write questions that require students to think about their own knowledge and experiences—for example, what are some reasons why each story had a different ending? What were the factors that made for failure or success?
10. Give your work to the teacher to check so that you can revise it if necessary.
11. Distribute copies of the stories to the class. Each group member takes a turn reading and asking classmates the discussion questions.

Project #4—How Can You Tell If Someone Is an Alcoholic?

Introduction
Amy isn't sure whether or not Takashi is an alcoholic, and neither is the doctor. How do you know when someone is an alcoholic or addicted?

Task
Your task is to make a poster with information to help people to decide when it might be important to seek help for problems with alcohol.

Skills
Critical thinking, research, note taking, working in a group, making presentations

Process
1. Review the case study.
2. Discuss the following in a group: Does anyone in the group know someone who is an alcoholic? Does anyone have training or work experience with people who are alcoholics? Share knowledge with the group.
3. Have group members share ideas on how they might begin to determine if someone has a problem with alcoholism. How do you know when you have had too much to drink and are drunk? Talk about the problem of alcoholism in your state and in your country. Is it a big problem?
4. Go to the Project Care website *(http://projectcare.worlded.org/alcoholism/ information.html#project4)*. You will find helpful information that you can use in your project.
5. Make discussion questions to ask the class. Make questions that ask students to share their own knowledge, experiences, and opinions.
6. Make a poster. Each student makes a section of the poster.
7. Give your work to the teacher to check so that you can revise it if necessary.
8. Present the poster to the class.

Reflection

Review the activities in this unit, and then evaluate your progress by answering the questions.

What did you learn about...

- **English**—How did you improve in the areas of reading, writing, speaking, or listening? List two new words or grammar points that you learned.

_____

_____

_____

_____

- **Health**—What did you learn about alcoholism or alcohol abuse? List at least two new things you learned.

_____

_____

_____

_____

- **Caregiving**—What did you learn about how you can help others? List at least two new things you learned about how you can help a person with a drinking problem.

_____

_____

_____

_____

Moving On

What do you need or want to learn more about?

_____

_____

_____

_____

_____

Can you think of ways that you can apply what you learned in this unit to your life or job?

_____

_____

_____

_____

_____

Your Health Care Dictionary

List the vocabulary words and expressions you learned that are related to health care. Write a definition or synonym next to each. Then write a sentence that uses the word.

1.

_____

_____

2.

_____

_____

3.

_____

_____

4.

_____

_____

5.

_____

_____

6.

_____

_____

7.

_____

_____

8.

_____

_____

9.

_____

_____

10.

_____

_____

11.

_____

_____

12.

_____

_____

Is It the Aging Process or Alzheimer's Disease?

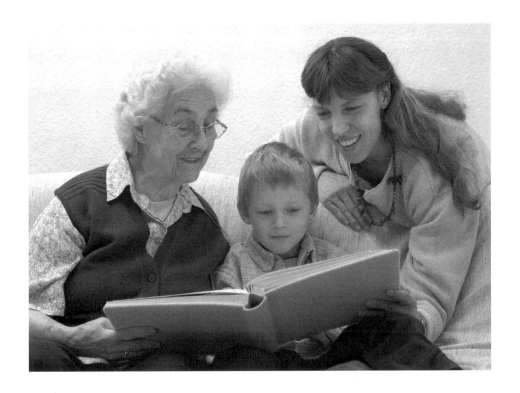

Imagining with Images

Imagine you are talking to the older woman in the picture. She tells you the same story over and over, and sometimes she repeats her questions. What does this make you think about her?

Before You Begin

What Vocabulary Do You Already Know?

Some of the words related to this topic that you may hear in your work or in discussions with health professionals are listed. You will find these words used in this unit. How many do you already know? As you complete the unit and learn the meanings of these words and phrases, add them to Your Health Care Dictionary pages at the end of the unit.

activities of daily living

ambulatory

around-the-clock care

assisted care facility/assisted caregiver

brain disorder

cognitive/cognition

deterioration

early stage/early onset

incontinence

live on [one's] own

long-term care (facility)

nursing home

retirement community/home

What Do You Already Know about This Topic?

1. Put a check mark next to the phrases you think are true about most older people. In a small group, talk about your answers.

   Most older people...

   ☐ have close contact with family.

   ☐ are almost all alike.

   ☐ are sick, weak, and dependent on others.

   ☐ have difficulty thinking clearly.

   ☐ are depressed.

   ☐ have personality changes, and they become more difficult to deal with as they get older.

   ☐ successfully adjust to the difficulties of getting old.

Now compare your group's answers with the information from the American Psychological Association. Notice that only two are true. You should have checked only the first and last boxes.

Most older people...

- ☑ have close contact with family.
- ☐ are almost all alike.
- ☐ are sick, weak, and dependent on others.
- ☐ have difficulty thinking clearly.
- ☐ are depressed.
- ☐ have personality changes, and they become more difficult to deal with as they get older.
- ☑ successfully adjust to the difficulties of getting old.

2. Answer the following questions. If you feel comfortable and if your teacher asks, talk about your answers with another student.

   - We all forget things at times. When is forgetting normal and when is it a serious problem?

   _____

   _____

   - Forgetting is common in older people, but sometimes it can be one symptom of a serious disease called Alzheimer's. Do you know what Alzheimer's disease is?

   _____

   _____

   - Do you know any older people who need someone to help take care of them? Give examples of the type of help these people need. Who is taking care of them?

   _____

   _____

Previewing the Case Study

What You Need to Know

Preparing to Read the Case Study

Preview the reading about the health topic and the case study. Read about the topic to help you get a better understanding of the vocabulary and issues associated with Alzheimer's disease. Important health care-related terms and phrases are in **bold** type. Then read a summary of the case study. Some of the vocabulary words that are in color in the case study are often-used English words that are helpful in many situations. How many of the **bold** or color words/phrases do you already know?

INTERACT ONLINE»

:: Go to *http://projectcare.worlded.org/alzheimers/case.html* to listen to the summary of the case study.

What is Alzheimer's? Alzheimer's disease (AD) is a **brain disorder** that affects people's ability to perform **activities of daily living.**

What causes it? Doctors don't know the exact cause of AD, but a collection of certain chemicals in the brain and the death of brain cells seem to be involved. A person's age and family history are factors. After the age of 65, the number of people with Alzheimer's disease increases significantly. Genetics might play a part in some forms of Alzheimer's disease.

What are its symptoms? Forgetfulness is usually the first symptom noticed. It starts to interfere with the ability to perform routine tasks and to live independently. People might forget words, names, dates, and where they left things. Later, they forget how to do simple things like using a television or driving a car. Still later, they forget how to dress or button their shirt. As the disease progresses, more **cognitive** and behavioral changes occur. For example, these people might have difficulty speaking, writing, reading, and understanding. They don't recognize people and places they know. They sometimes become aggressive or nervous, or they wander and get lost. In the end, patients must have **around-the-clock care.**

SUMMARY OF THE CASE STUDY

Mary Casey is a polite, energetic 80-year-old widow. Mary is in good health except that there is some **deterioration** of her memory. Recently there was an incident where she wandered away from her house and got lost. After an examination, a doctor found evidence of Alzheimer's disease. Mary has been **living on her own** now for two years and reports that she enjoys being independent. Sometime in the near future, however, she will need help so she can cope with **activities of daily living** around the house. Her two sons, Sam and Bob, are both thinking about asking their mother to live with them.

Vocabulary Check

Definitions of color words used in the unit follow. Review the definitions to check your understanding of the words and how they are used in the unit.

administer *(verb)* — to give

burden *(noun)* — an extra responsibility, a problem

chore *(noun)* — a necessary task (not fun)

cope with *(verb)* — to face a problem and overcome it

evaluate *(verb)* — to study and make a judgment about

evidence *(noun)* — words or objects that support the truth; proof

genetics *(noun)* — scientific study of the passing of characteristics from parents to children

insist *(verb)* — to demand

interfere *(verb)* — to prevent or disrupt something

priority *(noun)* — tasks or beliefs that are the most important

progress *(verb)* — to advance or become better or worse

realistic *(adjective)* — practical

routine *(noun)* — a series of things someone does regularly

support *(verb)* — to help

wander *(verb)* — to go from place to place without a plan

widow *(noun)* — a wife whose husband has died

Case Study

Mary Casey

Mary Casey is an 82-year-old widow who **lives on her own** in the house she once shared with her husband. Mary's younger son Sam is an auto mechanic. After his father died, he moved to a small third-floor apartment closer to his mother. Bob, Mary's older son, is a computer engineer. He and his wife Sara are expecting their first baby. They live in another state in a new four-bedroom home.

Last year, Mary Casey's family began to notice that she was having problems with her memory. At first they didn't think it was a problem because they knew it is common for many older people to have difficulty remembering names and where the keys are sometimes. Initially, Mary admitted that she was forgetting some simple things. As time passed, Mary's family and friends noticed that she often asked the same question over and over. They also could see that Mary was not taking care of herself like she had previously. Her appearance was **deteriorating,** and she was wearing the same clothes day after day. Her sons discovered that she hadn't been remembering to mail her bills. After Mary walked into the street late one night and was found wandering around the neighborhood by the police, Sam convinced his mother to see a doctor. The family was relieved that at last a trained professional would evaluate their mother.

A Diagnosis?

Mary's primary care physician gave her a thorough examination, but he was not able to decide whether Mary was just adjusting to aging or if there was something else wrong with her.

He referred her to a specialist, Dr. Laura Sosa. Dr. Sosa administered a number of tests to Mary. When the results came in, she called Mary and her family to her office for a conference.

Dr. Sosa explained that the test results indicated that Mary had Alzheimer's disease. In the conference with Mary and Sam, she explained that she had found evidence of serious changes in the brain and its ability to function. It was clear that Alzheimer's was the source of the problems with her memory.

Prognosis

Dr. Sosa gave her prognosis, explaining that the disease was in a moderate stage. Mary admitted that it was true that the activities she does regularly, such as shopping, cooking, and balancing her checkbook, were hard for her. The doctor nodded and added that, depending on how fast the disease progresses, even recalling names of family members will become more difficult.

Dr. Sosa talked about some ways Mary and the family could cope with her problems. She prescribed medications that might slow the progress of the disease. Dr. Sosa recommended that the family meet with a specialist to learn how to make daily life easier for everyone. She explained that additional help with daily activities would be needed. The doctor was concerned about Mary living in her house alone and recommended that the family have a meeting about how they can help keep her safe. Dr. Sosa's prognosis was that it was presently too challenging for Mary to care for herself and soon she would need **around-the-clock care.**

Understanding the Case Study

Answer each question about the case study. Use complete sentences.

1. What disease does Mary Casey have? How has the disease affected Mary's life?

   _____

   _____

2. Why didn't Sam call the doctor sooner?

   _____

   _____

3. Who was invited to the conference with Dr. Sosa? Why?

   _____

   _____

4. What is the prognosis for Mary?

   _____

   _____

5. Dr. Sosa suggested one way that Mary could help cope with her memory problems. What suggestion did the doctor give to Mary?

   _____

   _____

   _____

6. How will Mary's disease affect the rest of her family?

_____

_____

7. What do you think will happen to Mary? Where will she live?

_____

_____

Caring for Someone Who Has Alzheimer's

In the past, both of Mary's sons have talked to her about her living with them. But Mary has always **insisted** on **living on her own.** She loves her neighborhood and has many friends her age. She enjoys her independence and the control she has over her own life. Mary has also explained that she does not want to be a **burden** on her children. Although she has begun to accept help with some **chores** around the house occasionally, she wants to remain as independent as she can for as long as she can. She has made it very clear that she never wants to be put in a **nursing home.**

Sam and Bob talk about their mother's diagnosis. Sam proposes that Mary stay with him, but Bob and Sara think that he is not being **realistic.** Although he can always exchange the couch in the living room for another bed, his apartment is too small. He also works during the day, and so he is unable to stay home with her. Moreover, **around-the-clock nursing care** for Mary will not be possible on his salary as a mechanic.

Sam disagrees. He points out that if his mother stays with him, she will remain near her friends. He also thinks that maybe some of her friends could help out at times. He knows that friends are important to Mary and her overall health.

Bob says that he thinks she should live with her family. However, he knows that Mary could get good care in a **retirement community** with **assisted care.** He knows that they cannot afford that type of care. He has much more room than Sam does, so he offers for their mother to stay with his wife and him.

Sam asks Bob if he has thought about the stress that comes with a new baby. This, on top of caring for someone with Alzheimer's, can be very difficult. He wonders if that stress will be good for their mother. Sara agrees and seems surprised that Bob has not spoken with her about his idea first. She read that it can be very hard to supervise someone with Alzheimer's, and, for example, that people with this disease can do things like forget to turn off the stove. Sara feels that it might be too dangerous for the new baby. She says she will try to support Bob but admits that this isn't the best time to take his mother in. She would like to care for her mother-in-law, but also feels strongly that their baby's safety has to be their first priority.

Increasing Your Understanding

Group Work

Complete the chart. Work with a partner. List which aspects of the disease you think will be especially challenging for Mary and her family to handle.

Challenges for Mary and Her Family

Discussion—What Should Sam and Bob Do?

Work in small groups. Imagine you are related to Mary. What would you do? Use some of the phrases given.

Suggesting Action and Giving Advice
You **could** take some….
She **might (not)** want to think about attending….
If I were you, I'd….
He **should (not)** try….
You **ought to** go….
They **had better** start….
We **(do not) have** to….
They **must** give….
Why don't you….
Whatever you do, don't….

Talk about all the possible options for Mary. Decide as a group which ones are realistic. Try to decide as a group what you think is the best plan for Mary. If you cannot make a decision, discuss why you think it is hard for a family to make such decisions about an older parent.

Learning More about the Topic*

According to the Alzheimer's Association, there are more than 5 million people in the United States with Alzheimer's disease. Most of these people are over the age of 65. Those with **early-onset** Alzheimer's are under age 65.

There is no known cure for Alzheimer's, and no treatment can stop it. Researchers are learning more about this disease every year. There are drugs that can slow its progress. Some health care professionals feel that the risk of getting Alzheimer's can be reduced by doing things that help stimulate the mind. This includes playing chess, doing crossword puzzles, exercising, and interacting with friends and family.

---

*Although the information in this book might be helpful, it does not replace professional advice for individual cases. You should consult a health professional if you or a loved one has a serious illness.

Even if family members want to keep a person with Alzheimer's disease in their home, they may eventually need someone who can supervise the person's activities and keep him or her safe. They may also need counseling for the Alzheimer's person and the family, and the person with Alzheimer's may need treatment for other related problems such as depression. He or she may even wander away from the home, risking serious injury or death. Over time, the individual will become incontinent and will not be able to remember to eat or drink, will not be able to stand or sit, and will be unable to get out of bed.

When a person with Alzheimer's can no longer live alone or in a retirement community that does not offer 24/7 care, family members have to move the person into an assisted care facility or nursing home. These long-term care facilities specialize in taking care of patients who have diseases like Alzheimer's or who are no longer ambulatory. People with Alzheimer's die an average of four to six years after diagnosis, but the disease can last from three to 20 years.

Learning More from an Expert: Video

INTERACT ONLINE»

:: Go to *http://projectcare.worlded.org/alzheimers/video.html* to watch a video about Alzheimer's. You will hear a professional giving an opinion about what Mary's family can do to help her. Before you watch you might want to review some vocabulary used in the video at *http://projectcare.worlded.org/alzheimers/vocab.html*. After you complete the listening activity, do the activity below as part of a group or independently.

Discuss/Write

1. Do you agree with the expert's advice? Why or why not?

2. Considering what you have learned so far in this unit, what do you think are the most important steps Mary's family should take?

Writing

Give your opinion by answering each question in a well-developed paragraph.

1. What would you do if you and your parents lived near each other and one of them had a serious medical problem that required 24-hour care?

_____

_____

_____

_____

_____

_____

_____

_____

_____

_____

_____

_____

_____

_____

_____

_____

_____

_____

2. Would you make the same decision about your parents if you lived in a country other than the United States? Why or why not?

_____

_____

_____

_____

_____

_____

_____

_____

_____

_____

_____

_____

_____

_____

_____

_____

_____

_____

_____

_____

Projects

There are many people with Alzheimer's, and it is predicted that 14 million Americans will have the disease by 2050. Learn all you can about Alzheimer's and how you can help others. The projects will help improve your English conversation, writing, and reading skills and help you prepare yourself and your classmates to support someone with Alzheimer's disease.

INTERACT ONLINE»

:: The following projects were designed so that you can go to the Internet and other resources to find more information about Alzheimer's disease and how to care for people who have it. You and your teacher may use a checklist to evaluate your work. To find updated links to health information and checklists that will help you with your projects, go to the Project Care website at *http://projectcare.worlded.org/ alzheimers/projects.html*.

Project #1—Caregiver's Brochure

Introduction
When a person develops Alzheimer's disease as Mary has, it is often difficult for the family to take care of her or him. Dr. Sosa explained in the case study some of the cognitive and behavioral changes that will occur. What information do the family members need so they can take care of their loved one in the best way possible?

Task
Your task is to create a caregiver's guide (brochure or video) for families taking care of family members with Alzheimer's. Although you can include some basic information about the disease, you should focus on how friends and family can help. Make sure that you also include how the caregivers can take care of themselves.

Skills
Critical thinking, research, writing, acting, working in groups, making presentations

Process
1. Make sure you read and understand the instructions before you begin working on your project.
2. Find out if anyone in the group has experience with people who have Alzheimer's and ask him or her to share knowledge with the group.
3. Using what you learned from the reading, talk about the symptoms people with Alzheimer's experience.
4. Then list concerns family members probably have about taking care of a person with these symptoms. For example, "She might wander away and get lost."
5. Add more concerns to your group's list. Go to the Project Care website (*http://projectcare.worlded.org/alzheimers/information.html#project1*). You will find helpful information that you can use in your project by clicking on the link to Planning for Alzheimer's Care.
6. Or you can find books, magazine, or newspaper articles at the library, or talk to people with experience working with people who have Alzheimer's.
7. Have each student choose one area of concern from the group's list to research.
8. Find suggestions on how to handle your area of concern. For example, "You might need to get her 24-hour care." Some possible resources include:
   a. *http://projectcare.worlded.org/alzheimers/information.html#project1*. Click on the link to Caring for Someone with Alzheimer's.
   b. Interview health professionals at a nearby hospital (in person or by telephone).
   c. Find newspaper or magazine articles, or books at your local library.
9. Have each group member write the following for the caregiver's guide:
   a. the area of concern
   b. suggestions for help with the area of concern

10. Meet and read what each other wrote. Give each other suggestions for revision—what do you like? What is clear? What is confusing? Edit your stories before creating a final version to give to your teacher.

11. Create a guide (booklet or video) with information from all group members. (Microsoft Word has a template for a brochure.) For those making a brochure: Each student types his or her section. For those making a video: Each student takes a turn videotaping and being videotaped, giving information about his or her area of research.

12. Give your work to the teacher to check so that you can revise it if necessary.

13. Present the booklet or video to the class.

Project #2—What's the Latest News?

Introduction
Health professionals have been learning more about Alzheimer's in recent years. What is the current information about the disease and treatments for it?

Task
Your task is to make a poster about current information and treatments for Alzheimer's.

Skills
Critical thinking, research, working in groups, graphic design, making presentations

Process
1. Review the case study.
2. Find out if anyone in the group has experience with people who have Alzheimer's? Share knowledge with the group.
3. Have each student get information about a different aspect. Decide with your group which aspect each member will research:
   a. cause of the disease
   b. symptoms of the disease
   c. treatments
   d. what health professionals think they may know in the near future
   e. research information.
   Go to the Project Care website
   (http://projectcare.worlded.org/alzheimers/information.html#project2).
   You will find helpful information that you can use in your project.
4. Share information with your group.
5. Make a poster. Each student makes a section of the poster explaining the aspect of Alzheimer's she or he researched.
6. Give your work to the teacher to check so that you can revise it if necessary.
7. Present your poster to the class.

Project #3—Advice for Caregivers

Introduction

Wherever Mary ends up living, her family will be involved with her care and support. Caring for a person with Alzheimer's, however, can be very difficult. What are some of the difficulties for caregivers, and what can they do to make things easier?

Task

Your task is to develop a short training to help relatives and friends who care for people with Alzheimer's.

Skills

Critical thinking, research, communicating, giving advice and counseling others, working in groups, teaching, making presentations

Process

1. Review the case study, if needed.
2. Find out if anyone in the group has experience with people who have Alzheimer's? Share knowledge with the group.
3. Go to the Project Care website *(http://projectcare.worlded.org/alzheimers/ information.html#project3)*. You will find helpful information that you can use in your project.
4. Make a list of the difficulties that caregivers can have when taking care of people with Alzheimer's.
5. Have each student choose at least one difficulty to research. Find out why it occurs, and how a person can cope with it.
6. Have each student prepare a presentation for the class on what she or he researched. Include images and written information.
7. Practice your presentation, and give each other feedback.
8. Have your teacher view your presentation to check so that you can revise it if necessary.
9. Present to the class.

Project #4—Acting It Out

Introduction
Mary and her family each have a different point of view on the situation. Imagine that Mary, her family, and doctor have a meeting together. What does each person say in the meeting? At the end of the meeting, what is their decision about Mary's care?

Task
Write and then act out a drama for the class about what happens in the meeting, and the decision they make.

Skills
Critical thinking, research, acting, writing, working in groups, making presentations

Process
1. Review the case study.
2. Find out if anyone in the group has experience with people who have Alzheimer's? Share knowledge with the group.
3. Go to the Project Care website *(http://projectcare.worlded.org/alzheimers/ information.html#project4)*. You will find helpful information that you can use in your project.
4. Discuss each person's point of view:
   a. Mary
   b. Sam
   c. Bob
   d. Sara
   e. Dr. Sosa
5. Have each student choose one person to role play.
6. Act out the meeting two or three times. Make the discussion different each time to see which points, opinions, and other factors are most important to include in your final drama.
7. Discuss how to organize the drama. Each student writes his or her part, and gives it to one student who puts the parts together in written form, making sure each person has equal opportunity to speak in the drama. Distribute the drama to the group members.
8. Meet and read what each other wrote. Give each other suggestions for revision—what do you like? What is clear? What is confusing? Edit your stories and create a final version to give to your teacher.
9. Practice the drama.
10. Have your teacher observe your practice to check so that you can revise it if necessary.
11. Perform the drama for the class. Ask the class to give their reactions. Tell the class about the process of making the drama: any agreement, disagreements, and important or interesting points discussed while creating the drama.

Reflection

Review the activities in this unit, and then evaluate your progress by answering the questions.

What did you learn about...

- **English**—How did you improve in the areas of reading, writing, speaking, or listening? List at least two new words or grammar points that you learned.

  _____

  _____

  _____

  _____

- **Health**—What did you learn about Alzheimer's or the health field in general? List at least two new things you learned.

  _____

  _____

  _____

  _____

- **Caregiving**—What did you learn about how you can help others? List at least two new things you learned about how you can help a person with Alzheimer's.

  _____

  _____

  _____

  _____

Moving On

What do you need or want to learn more about?

_____

_____

_____

_____

_____

Can you think of ways that you can apply what you learned in this unit to your life or job?

_____

_____

_____

_____

_____

Your Health Care Dictionary

List the vocabulary words and expressions you learned that are related to health care. Write a definition or synonym next to each. Then write a sentence that uses the word.

1.

_____

_____

2.

_____

_____

3.

_____

_____

4.

_____

_____

5.

_____

_____

6.

_____

_____

7.

_____

_____

8.

_____

_____

9.

_____

_____

10.

_____

_____

11.

_____

_____

12.

_____

_____

13.

_____

_____

14.

_____

_____

15.

_____

_____

16.

_____

_____

17.

_____

_____

18.

_____

_____

19.

_____

_____

When Is It Time to Let Go?

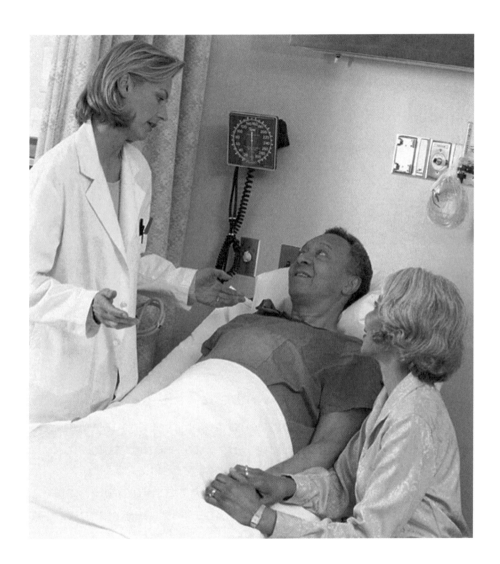

Imagining with Images

Imagine you are visiting the man in the picture. He is a friend or relative, and he is going to die soon. What would you say to him? What do you think he wants to talk about?

Before You Begin

What Vocabulary Do You Already Know?

Some of the words related to this topic that you may hear in your work or in discussions with health professionals are listed. You will find these words used in this unit. How many do you already know? As you complete the unit and learn the meanings of these words and phrases, add them to Your Health Care Dictionary pages at the end of the unit.

bed-ridden	hospice
bereavement counselors	impending death
chemotherapy/chemo	oncology/oncologist
coma	palliative care
consciousness	regimen
end stage	terminal illness
grief cycle/counseling	to be terminally ill
grieving period	

What Do You Already Know about This Topic?

Write your answers to the questions. If you feel comfortable and if your teacher asks, talk about your answers with another student.

1. Has anyone close to you died? If you are comfortable, share your experience with one other person in the class. If you prefer not to talk about it, write about it instead.

_____

_____

2. Give your opinion of these common ideas about someone who is dying. Do you agree or disagree? What has been your experience? Discuss with a classmate.

A. Most people who are dying don't want to talk about it.

_____

_____

_____

B. When people are near death, they usually want all their friends to be around them.

_____

_____

_____

C. Most people want the doctor to tell them if they are going to die.

_____

_____

_____

D. While dying, people see a white light, a tunnel.

_____

_____

_____

Here are some comments from some experts who help people through the dying process in the United States. Please keep in mind that when preparing to die, each individual's experiences or wishes vary from person to person and culture to culture.

1. "A person may want to openly discuss his or her illness and **impending death,** or he or she may avoid discussing it. The key is to follow your friend's lead. Keep in mind that your friend will experience this illness in his or her own unique way." *(Hospice Net)*

2. "The person may only want to be with a very few or even just one person. This is a sign of preparation for release from the person/people whom the support is most needed in order to make the transition. If you are not part of this inner circle at the end, it does not mean you are not loved or are unimportant. It means you have already done what your loved one asked of you, and it is the time for you to say good-bye. If you are part of the final inner circle of support, the person needs your support and permission to let go." *(Hospice Net)*

3. "Because studies show that a majority of patients want to discuss prognosis, it is recommended that physicians ask how patients want to talk about prognosis. Because many patients may not understand the term *prognosis,* an alternative is to ask, 'How much do you want to know about the likely course of this illness?' These questions require response that goes beyond a yes or no answer. There is also a range of options: Some people want lots of details, some want the big picture, and others prefer that a doctor talk to their family." *(Journal of Clinical Oncology)*

4. "In general, this is not true. As people die there are physical and chemical changes in the brain that result in a gradual loss of **consciousness.** Some people experience something similar to dreaming while still awake. Some persons say they see relatives who have previously died. In almost all instances, these last visions are usually pleasant and offer comfort to the dying person, especially regarding the possibility of reuniting with deceased loved ones." *(Hospice Foundation of America)*

Previewing the Case Study

What You Need to Know

Preparing to Read the Case Study

Preview the reading about the health topic and the case study. Read about the topic to help you get a better understanding of the vocabulary and issues associated with death. Important health care-related terms and phrases are in **bold** type. Then read a summary of the case study. Some of the vocabulary words that are in color in the case study are often-used English words that are helpful in many situations. How many of the **bold** or color words/phrases do you already know?

INTERACT ONLINE»

:: Go to *http://projectcare.worlded.org/dying/case.html* to listen to the summary of the case study.

Dying is a process that occurs when the body slows down its systems. This process is different for each person. In general, the person's desire for food decreases as weakness and sleepiness increase. A change in body functions, such as digestion, will occur. Some people slip into a **coma** before dying. An exact time of death cannot be predicted, nor can the exact way a person will die.

To care properly for a dying person, a caregiver—whether a family member or not—must understand the specific disease or condition and its effect on the person. Does the person have pain and/or other symptoms of discomfort? Is the person **bed-ridden** ("non-ambulatory")? Does the person have special medical and nutritional needs? Is the person fully or only partly **conscious**? Is the person in the **end stage** of the illness? Can the person communicate his or her needs?

SUMMARY OF THE CASE STUDY

Alex Moskovin is battling cancer. His **oncologist** in-
formed him that he was in an advanced stage of lung
cancer and it was necessary to submit to another **regimen** of **chemotherapy.** Alex let the information sink in
and said that he would think about whether or not to
continue treatment. Even though his sister, Natasha,
wanted to talk about this decision, Alex avoided any
discussion of it for a while. As time passed, Alex began
to hint that he might not want to undergo more treatment and talked about **palliative care** and **hospice.** He
wondered if going through **chemotherapy** was futile
and mentioned that he didn't want to risk dying in a
medical facility. Natasha sensed Alex was ready to tell
her about his decision, but she wasn't sure how she
should respond.

Vocabulary Check

Definitions of the color words used in the unit follow. Review the definitions to check your understanding of the words and how they are
used in the unit.

anticipate *(verb)* — to expect

bargain *(verb)* — to negotiate or strike a deal

bias *(noun)* — general belief in favor of or against something

burden *(verb)* — to cause trouble or extra effort

denial *(noun)* — rejection

dilemma *(noun)* — a difficult choice usually between two alternatives

disconcerting *(adjective)* — disturbing, unsettling

dull *(verb)* — to make less sharp or intense

futile *(adjective)* — not worth attempting, useless

get to the point *(idiom)* — say what's important

grueling *(adjective)* — very difficult and tiring

hint *(verb)* — to make reference to something indirectly

nutrition *(noun)* — the study of how the body needs and uses food

predict *(verb)* — to say what will happen in the future

resolve *(verb)* — to decide to do something

sink in (idiom) — to gradually understand

submit *(verb)* — to agree to

torture *(noun)* — physical abuse that causes pain and mental stress

withdrawn *(adjective)* — quiet, not communicating

Case Study

Alex Moskovin

Alex Moskovin is a 56-year-old teacher who has been battling lung cancer for years. He came from Russia to New York City with his only sister, Natasha. She is a single mother and lives with her two young daughters.

Although Natasha is younger than Alex, they are very close. Alex has always helped his sister when she needed it, and now it is Natasha's turn to help him. As a way of coping with her feelings about her brother's **terminal illness,** she has been keeping a diary. Below are her diary entries.

August 30, 2006

This morning Alex got a call from his **oncologist** about his latest test results. Dr. Petrov wanted him to come to his office that afternoon. Alex knew it couldn't be good news since Dr. Petrov would have told him that on the phone.

Alex called me immediately. I knew the matter must have been serious because he was very **conscious** of not asking me to take off any more time from work than I already had.

As we walked in the door at the doctor's office, Dr. Petrov got up and walked around the desk to greet us. He asked us to sit in two large leather chairs in front. Dr. Petrov began by saying that he would get to the point. He told us that the test results weren't good.

He explained that the cancer in Alex's lungs has spread and that the latest **regimen** of **chemotherapy** didn't get it all. Doctor Petrov paused. Then he lowered his eyes and said, "I'm sorry." Asking the question I was sure the doctor was anticipating, I asked what else could be done. He explained that the cancer is at an advanced or **end stage,** and that submitting to more aggressive treatment could extend Alex's life for several months.

What Alex said then surprised me. He said in a soft voice that he'd have to give that some thought. Dr. Petrov nodded and said that although it is not very often that someone chooses to refuse treatment, Alex certainly has that right.

Sept. 2, 2006

A few days have passed now and still Alex has not spoken about whether to have more **"chemo"** or not. I'll wait a little bit longer, though I am starting to get frustrated. Isn't he afraid that the cancer is growing in him while he waits to make a decision? Or maybe he just wants to spend a few more days imagining that he is normal and "free of cancer" without having to think about going back for treatments. I want so much to talk this decision through with Alex and get this resolved. I realize that it is selfish of me, but his decision also affects me as well as my family.

Sept. 6, 2006

As time passed, I realized that maybe Alex didn't want to burden me by talking about his dilemma. Maybe he wanted me to ask him about it, so I did. It turned out he didn't want to discuss it at all! I tried to talk about it last night when we sat down to dinner after the kids went to bed. Alex slammed his glass down and said, "Could we just enjoy the meal?" But later that night, knowing I was upset, Alex apologized for getting angry. He explained that he wanted to avoid thinking about the topic altogether. He talked about how a man is supposed to be strong, but he admitted that he wasn't sure if he could handle any more **chemotherapy**. I have to admit that it was disconcerting. As my big brother, he has always been the one I looked to for support. In the end Alex promised that he would try to come to a decision soon.

Sept. 8, 2006

It is understandable that he is having a difficult time with this, but I have to confess that it has been torture for me, too. At least Alex and I are now talking more about the decision. He is considering all the information that we found during our recent research on the Internet. He goes back and forth. One day he discovers some new diet that might help and leans toward **chemotherapy.** Then the next day he decides against it. I don't think I am helping. I try to stay neutral, but my guess is that I show my bias.

Sept. 10, 2006

I can't stop wanting Alex to make the decision to live longer. I guess I am not ready to give up yet. Maybe the doctors are wrong. Or maybe there will be a new treatment soon. I know the treatments are grueling; yet, there might be some newer drugs that can dull the pain. I don't think I am being selfish if there might be a chance, as small as it is.

Sept. 15, 2006

Alex has seemed withdrawn and has not responded to my invitations to come over for dinner lately. Today when I called him he said something that upset me. He told me that no matter which decision he makes, he is still going to die sooner or later. It made me realize that the most important person in my life, except for my children, is doing to die. No matter what we do, it is only a few months that he'll be alive. He is my only relative here, and I don't know what I will do without his love and support. I don't want to write any more about this right now. I am just too sad.

Understanding the Case Study

Answer each question about the case study. Use complete sentences.

1. What kind of doctor is Dr. Petrov?

   _____

   _____

2. How long can Alex live if he chooses chemotherapy?

   _____

   _____

3. What did the doctor say and do in order to communicate how serious the situation was?

   _____

   _____

4. Why do you think Alex didn't want to think about his situation?

   _____

   _____

5. Even though Alex read a lot of information about cancer and treatments, why couldn't he decide what to do?

   _____

   _____

6. What made Natasha sad and want to stop writing in her diary?

   _____

   _____

7. Can you predict what Alex will decide to do? Explain why you think this.

_____

_____

Caring for Someone Who Is Going to Die

Sept. 21, 2006

Just in passing, Alex mentioned how he fears the possibility of dying in a hospital. He heard that many people die trying as many new treatments as they can in a futile attempt to fight off the disease. It seems that Alex is considering his alternatives, including **palliative care** and **hospice.**

He still hasn't said anything to me. I'm afraid to ask him about it because if he has decided to refuse treatment, I would have to accept the reality that he actually will die. I want him to live! I want him to keep fighting and not to quit. How many times has he told me that and helped me through tough times? Wouldn't that be what he would say to me? I know it isn't I who would have to suffer through the **chemo,** but maybe I should encourage him to try. But then again, I don't want him to do it just for me. I want to be supportive if Alex decides to refuse **chemotherapy,** but I don't know what I should say.

Increasing Your Understanding

Group Work

Sometimes in a course or at work you will be asked to write your thoughts or opinions on a topic and support them with examples and details. Below are some questions with incomplete answers. Discuss with a partner how you would complete the answers. Then in your own words, write at least one sentence to complete the thought and prove your point.

Question 1: When someone is facing death, he or she often first goes through the stage of denial. Please explain if you think Alex went though this stage, and if so, how did he experience it?

It seems that Alex Moskovin entered the stage of denial almost immediately after his appointment with Dr. Petrov. The clearest evidence of this is that...

_____

_____

_____

_____

Question 2: At some point during the process of preparing for death, it is normal that one feels and expresses anger about the situation. Please explain if you think Alex went though a stage of anger. Please prove this with examples.

It is hard to tell if Alex went through a stage of anger, but there was one event when he showed he was angry. This occurred when...

_____

_____

_____

_____

Question 3: Sadness and depression are generally to be expected during the process of dying. Please explain if you think Alex was depressed, and if so how did he experience/express it?

To make an accurate diagnosis one would need to gather more information. However, there are some signs that Alex was depressed. One indication is...

_____

_____

_____

_____

Discussion—What Should Natasha Do?

Discuss the questions in a small group.

1. Imagine that Alex tells Natasha that he is refusing treatment. What should Natasha say?

2. If she doesn't support his decision to refuse treatment, should Natasha tell Alex how she feels? Why or why not?

3. If you think Alex should continue with chemotherapy treatment, would you change your opinion:

   - if it would only extend his life for a few days to week?

   - if you knew it would cause him a great deal of pain and discomfort?

4. If you think it is okay for Alex to refuse chemotherapy treatment, would you change your opinion:

   - if it would not cause him any physical pain?

   - if it would extend his life for more than a year?

Learning More about the Topic*

Caring for the dying requires special knowledge and skill. **Hospices** and other care facilities take care of the emotional, physical, and psychological needs of the **terminally ill.** They provide **palliative care.** This is care with the goal of managing pain and other possible symptoms of discomfort that may accompany the dying process.

People respond to death based on their own personality, family support system, culture, and spiritual beliefs. Elisabeth Kübler-Ross, a psychiatrist who specialized in care of the dying, said that a **terminally ill** person also goes through a **grief cycle** that includes five stages: denial, anger, bargaining for more time, depression, and acceptance. According to Kübler-Ross, a dying person does not necessarily go through all five stages or experience them in this order, but he or she will generally experience at least some stages of the cycle.

It takes time and healing, even for caregivers who are not related to the dying person, to come to terms with loss. If you are a caregiver, it's important to stay emotionally, physically, and psychologically healthy. Surround yourself with supportive family and friends. Do the things you love. Exercise and eat a healthy diet. Remember too that once the person has died, you will experience some sort of grief. If you find yourself unable to cope, **bereavement** support groups, grief **counselors,** and therapists are available to help you care for yourself.

---

*Although the information in this book might be helpful, it does not replace professional advice for individual cases. You should consult a health professional if you or a loved one has a serious illness.

Learning More from an Expert: Video

INTERACT ONLINE»

:: Go to *http://projectcare.worlded.org/dying/video.html* to watch a video about death and dying. You will hear a professional giving an opinion about what Natasha can do to help her brother. Before you watch, you might want to review some vocabulary used in the video at *http://projectcare.worlded.org/dying/vocab.html*. After you complete the listening activity, do the activity below as part of a group or independently.

Discuss/Write

1. Do you agree with the expert's advice? Why or why not?

2. Considering what you have learned so far in this unit, what do you think are the most important steps Natasha should take?

Writing

Give your opinion by answering each question in a well-developed paragraph.

1. What would most people from your culture do if a family member were dying and decided to stop treatment?

_____

_____

_____

_____

_____

_____

_____

_____

_____

2. What do you think helps people deal with death? What are the things that people can do to help someone they love who is dying?

_____

_____

_____

_____

_____

_____

_____

_____

_____

_____

_____

_____

_____

_____

_____

_____

_____

Projects

Everyone handles the topic of death and dying somewhat differently. Even though there are some typical stages, not everyone reacts in the same way. This is true whether one is talking about the person who is dying or the family and friends. This makes it hard to know the best way a caregiver can help. Nevertheless, the more we learn about the issues involved in the dying process, the more peace we might bring to others who face it. The projects will help improve your English conversation, writing, and reading skills and help you prepare yourself and your classmates to support someone who is dying.

INTERACT ONLINE»

:: The following projects were designed so that you can go to the Internet and other resources to find more information about the dying process and how to care for people dealing with it. You and your teacher may use a checklist to evaluate your work. To find updated links to health information and checklists that will help you with your projects, go to the Project Care website at *http://projectcare. worlded.org/dying/projects.html*.

Project #1—Information about and Support through the Dying Process

Introduction
Going through the process of dying usually isn't easy for the person who is dying. It's also difficult for his and her loved ones, before, during, and after the person dies. They can feel a little better if they have some information about the process of dying and grief.

Task
Your task is to make a guide for dying people and their loved ones to help them get through their experiences. Include information for the dying person, as well as for loved ones before, during, and after the person dies.

Skills
Writing, working on computers, graphic design

Process
1. Review the case study, if needed.
2. Find out if anyone in the group has information that can help people who are dying or their loved ones? Share knowledge with the group.
3. Make a list of difficulties (and positive experiences as well) that can occur for dying people and their friends and family.
4. Divide up the group so each person researches a different resource. Make sure the group covers information for a person who is dying as well as information for their loved ones. Go to the Project Care website *(http://projectcare.worlded. org/dying/information.html#project1)*. You will find helpful information that you can use in your project.
5. With your group, share the information that you have researched.
6. Have each student write a section for the guide. Look over each student's writing, giving feedback and making suggestions if needed. Give the first version to your teacher so he or she can review it.
7. Have students type up their sections, and have one student put them together into one guide. (Some word processors have templates for brochures.)
8. Have the group make up questions to ask the class after the presentations to help students test what they have learned about each topic. (For example: What is one thing you can do to help someone caring for a dying person?)
9. Class presentation: Distribute guides to the class. Each group member explains his or her section to the class. Ask the class the questions the group made up.

Project #2—Ending with Hospice

Introduction

When doctors determine that nothing more can be done to cure an illness, they might suggest hospice. Hospice is not a place but a kind of care that people can receive in a nursing facility or their homes. The idea of hospice care is to make the dying person as comfortable as possible in a familiar environment, with family and friends.

Task

Imagine that Alex decides to have hospice. Your task is to write the ending to the family's story. Learn what hospice care is and create a story that explains what hospice care might be like for Alex. You can choose to write this as a story, a diary, or a newspaper article.

Skills

Writing, reading, working on computers

Process

1. Review the case study if needed.
2. Learn more about hospice. Have each student in your group read a different resource. Go to the Project Care website *http://projectcare.worlded.org/ dying/information.html#project2)*. You will find helpful information that you can use in your project.
3. With your group, share the information you have researched.
4. Together with your group, list reasons family members may have for and against having hospice and discuss these.
5. With your group, write a possible ending to Alex and his family's story. The group can write several endings. Students may decide to work independently.
6. If students work independently to write different endings, share your endings with the group. Group members offer suggestions for revisions. Give your work to the teacher for review. Complete your final revision.
7. Present the story ending(s) to the class. Ask the class to give their reactions. Ask if they think they are realistic, and if they would have imagined a similar ending or not, and why.

Project #3—Write a Poem, Song, or Letter to Someone Who Is Dying

Introduction
There are many ways to express oneself to a loved one who is dying. What would you like to say?

Task
Imagine that someone you care for is dying. Write a poem, song, or letter to him or her.

Skills
Writing, composing music, working on computers, reading

Process
1. Find out if anyone in the group has experience communicating with people who were dying? If students feel comfortable, share knowledge with the group.
2. Each group member can choose the mode she or he wants to express her- or himself: a poem, a song, or a letter.
3. Research information for people who are dying and their loved ones to increase your understanding. Divide up the group so each person researches a different resource. Go to the Project Care website *http://projectcare.worlded.org/ dying/information.html#project3)*. You will find helpful information that you can use in your project.
4. With your group, share the information you have researched.
5. Write your song, poem, or letter.
6. Give your work to the teacher to check and revise it if necessary.
7. Share your poem, letter, and/or song with the class. Ask the class to give their reactions.

Project #4—What Can I Say?

Introduction
It can be difficult to know how to talk with someone who is dying. You are going to help Natasha learn ways she can be supportive of her brother.

Task
Your task is to role-play conversations between Natasha and Alex.

Skills
Speaking, listening, writing

Process
1. Find out if students in the group have talked with people who are/were in the process of dying, so they can share their knowledge with the group.
2. Have each student research a different resource for ways to communicate with people who are dying. Decide with the group which resource each student will research. Go to the Project Care website *(http://projectcare.worlded.org/dying/information.html#project4)*. You will find helpful information that you can use in your project.
3. With your group, share the information that you have researched.
4. Have students pair up. Working together, each pair writes a dialogue between Alex and Natasha that includes suggestions learned from the group's research.
5. Have each student practice the role-play for the project group and get feedback. Does the dialogue sound realistic? Does it include suggestions from the research? Any grammar, vocabulary, or sentence structure corrections necessary? Make changes in the dialogue if necessary.
6. As a group, make up questions for the class to discuss after each pair's presentation. The questions could be ones that help the rest of the class notice effective communication. (For example, how did Natasha show that she understood what Alex was feeling?)
7. For each presentation for the class, introduce the topic and the situation. Then perform role-plays for the class. After each role play, ask the class the questions and explain any other information that was learned from research.

Reflection

Review the activities in this unit, and then evaluate your progress by answering the questions.

What did you learn about...

- **English**—How did you improve in the areas of reading, writing, speaking, or listening? List at least two new words or grammar points that you learned.

  _____

  _____

  _____

  _____

- **Health**—What did you learn about death and dying or the health field in general? List at least two new things you learned.

  _____

  _____

  _____

  _____

- **Caregiving**—What did you learn about how you can help others? List at least two new things you learned about how you can help a person who is dying.

  _____

  _____

  _____

  _____

Moving On

What do you need or want to learn more about?

_____

_____

_____

_____

_____

Can you think of ways that you can apply what you learned in this unit to your life or job?

_____

_____

_____

_____

_____

Your Health Care Dictionary

List the vocabulary words and expressions you learned that are related to this unit. Write a definition or synonym next to each. Then write a sentence that uses the word.

1.

_____

_____

2.

_____

_____

3.

_____

_____

4.

_____

_____

5.

_____

_____

6.

_____

_____

7.

_____

_____

8.

_____

_____

9.

_____

_____

10.

_____

_____

11.

_____

_____

12.

_____

_____

13.

_____

_____

14.

_____

_____

15.

_____

_____

16.

_____

_____

17.

_____

_____

18.

_____

_____

Appendix
Evaluation Checklists

Students can evaluate their work on the projects by using the following checklists. You might want to adapt them by using a scoring scale so they can assess how well they did, for example, on a scale of 1-4. Make sure you explain how you will distinguish a score of 4 versus a score of 2 or 3. We have found checklists to be more practical for student use although best practice in project-based learning often involves a rubric.

To create a checklist or rubric suited to your students' needs, go to *http://projectcare.worlded.org/resources.html#checklists*.

Group Work Checklist – Project	✓
Listening I listened carefully and tried to understand what others said.	
Respecting I respected others' ideas and supported their ideas and efforts.	
Questioning I asked questions when I needed to understand others' ideas better.	
Helping I offered help to others in the group.	
Decision-making I contributed to the decision-making of the group.	
Sharing I shared ideas and reported what I learned to the group.	
Participation I contributed to the project by working on it as hard as the other members of the group.	
On-Task Behavior When the group met to work on the project, I was not distracted from the work.	
How do you think you did? Your comments:	Total ____

Writing Checklist – Project	✓
Introduction I started my writing with something interesting to get the reader's attention and introduced the main topic.	
Focus on Topic I stayed on the topic, writing about one main idea supported by details and examples.	
Conclusion I included a conclusion summarizing the topic.	
Content Knowledge I showed readers that I understood the topic, making sure to include information about who, what, when, where, why, as necessary.	
Organization I presented information in a logical order.	
Capitalization and Punctuation I did not make many errors in capitalization or punctuation.	
Grammar and Spelling I did not make many errors in grammar or spelling.	
References I used quotes for information I got from other readings.	
Revision I used a dictionary to check spelling and asked someone to check my grammar.	
How do you think you did? Your comments:	Total ___

Presentation Checklist – Project	✓
Preparation I practiced for the presentation so I was prepared.	
Organization I wrote notes or an outline ahead of time and presented information in an organized way. My presentation had a beginning, middle, and end. I made the main ideas clear.	
Revision I used a dictionary to check spelling and asked someone to check my grammar for any written work.	
Content Knowledge I demonstrated that I understand the important aspects of the topic, for example who, what, when, where, and why. I showed clear evidence of research.	
Speak Fluently I used good intonation and rhythm; I didn't speak too quickly or too slowly.	
Speak Clearly I used a clear voice and correct pronunciation of most vocabulary.	
Communicate with the Audience I made eye contact, involved the audience, and allowed the audience to ask questions.	
How do you think you did? Your comments:	Total ——

Sources

To the Teacher: How to Use This Book
Folse, K. *Vocabulary Myths. Applying Second Language Research to Classroom Teaching*. Ann Arbor: University of Michigan Press, 2004.

Unit 1
Depression: You Don't Have to Feel This Way. Leawood, KS: American Academy of Family Physicians, April 2005.

"Perspectives in Disease Prevention and Health Promotion Suicide—United States, 1970-1980." *Morbidity and Mortality Weekly Report*, June 21, 1985, 34, no. 24: 353-57.

Strock, M. *Depression*. Bethesda, MD: National Institute of Mental Health Public Information and Communications Branch, 2000. NIH Publication No. 00-3561.

Unit 2
Alcohol Use and Abuse. Bethesda, MD: National Institute on Alcohol Abuse and Alcoholism, 2005.

American Psychiatric Association. *Diagnostic and Statistical Manual of Mental Disorders, Fourth Edition*. Washington, DC: American Psychiatric Association, 2000.

D'Onofrio, Gail, and Linda C. Degutis. "Screening and Brief Intervention in the Emergency Department." *Alcohol Research and Health* 28, no. 2 (2004-2005). Bethesda, MD: National Institute on Alcohol Abuse and Alcoholism.

FAQs for the General Public. Bethesda, MD: National Institute on Alcohol Abuse and Alcoholism, 2007.

New Year, Old Myths, New Fatalities. Bethesda, MD: National Institute on Alcohol Abuse and Alcoholism, 2006. NIH Publication No. 06-5639.

Unit 3

Basics of Alzheimer's: What It Is, and What You Can Do. Chicago: Alzheimer's Association, n.d.

Caregiver Stress: Respect Your Well-Being. Chicago: Alzheimer's Association, n.d.

Fact Sheet: Alzheimer's Disease. Chicago: Alzheimer's Association, 2007.

Older Adults' Health and Age-Related Changes: Reality Versus Myth. Washington, DC: American Psychological Association Office of Public Communications, April 1998.

Respite Care Guide: Finding What's Best for You. Chicago: Alzheimer's Association, 2007.

What Is Alzheimer's? Chicago: Alzheimer's Association, 2007.

Unit 4

Creagan, E. *Grief: A Mayo Clinic Doctor Confronts Painful Emotions.* Rochester, MN: Mayo Clinic, 2006.

End of Life: Caring for Your Dying Loved One. Rochester, MN: Mayo Clinic, 2007.

Tatelbaum, J. *After Caregiving Ends. Journeys* (newsletter of the Hospice Foundation of America) (April 2001).

What You Can Do to Be a Supportive Caregiver. Nashville, TN: HospiceNet, n.d.